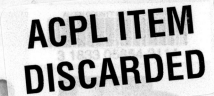

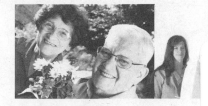
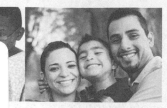

MANAGING YOUR MEDICARE:
An Insider's Guide to Maximizing Benefits and Lowering Costs

George Jacobs

Self-Counsel Press Inc.
(a subsidiary of)
International Self-Counsel Press Ltd.
USA   Canada

Library and Archives Canada Cataloguing in Publication

Jacobs, George

    Managing your medicare / George Jacobs.

ISBN 978-1-55180-857-4

1. National health services — United States. 2. Medical economics — United States. 3. Medical care, Cost of — United States. I. Title.

RA412.J32 2009   362.10973   C2009-902333-4

Cover and Inside Images
Copyright©iStockphoto/Senior: Happy Days/sdominick
Copyright©iStockphoto/Nurse Listening to Boy with Stethoscope/Photo Euphoria
Copyright©iStockphoto/Doctor/speedclimb
Copyright©iStockphoto/Young and elderly female/absolut_100
Copyright©iStockphoto/Loving family/aldomurillo

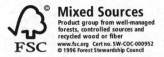

Mixed Sources
Product group from well-managed forests, controlled sources and recycled wood or fiber
FSC
www.fsc.org Cert no. SW-COC-000952
© 1996 Forest Stewardship Council

Self-Counsel Press Inc.
(a subsidiary of)
International Self-Counsel Press Ltd.

1704 North State Street   1481 Charlotte Road
Bellingham, WA 98225   North Vancouver, BC V7J 1H1
USA   Canada

CONTENTS

Introduction		xiii
1. Understanding The Basics of Enrollment in and Entitlement to Medicare's Programs		1
1. What is Medicare?		1
2. Medicare's Fundamental Programs		1
3. Entitlement		3
3.1 Entitlement based on a retirement account		3
3.2 Entitlement based on a survivor's account		5
3.3 Entitlement based on a disability account		6
3.4 Entitlement based on end-stage renal disease		7
3.5 Retroactive Part A entitlement		9
4. Buying into Medicare: Premium Part A		9
5. Enrollment Periods		11
5.1 Individual enrollment periods		12
5.2 General enrollment periods		12
5.3 Employer and union group health special enrollment period		13
5.4 Foreign situations		13
5.5 International volunteers		14
6. How Part B Coordinates with Your Other Health Insurance		14
7. Noncoverage outside the US		15

	8.	Getting Help Paying Your Part B Premium	16
	8.1	The Social Security savings clause	16
	8.2	Medicaid	16
	8.3	Medicare Savings Program	16
	8.4	Payment by employer, union, or other organization	17
	8.5	Reimbursement programs	17
	8.6	Your Medicare Advantage Part C health plan	19
	9.	Part B: High-Income Premium Surcharges	19
	9.1	Modified Adjusted Gross Income (MAGI)	20
	9.2	Requesting a change in premium surcharge	20
	9.3	Paying your premium amounts	23
	10.	Information about Your Medicare Number and Card	23

2 Part A — 25

	1.	Hospital Inpatient Stays	25
	1.1	Benefit period for inpatient stays	26
	1.2	Medicare hospital benefits	26
	1.3	Special notes on Medicare hospital coverage	27
	2.	Skilled Nursing Facility (SNF) Care	28
	2.1	Qualifying for a stay	28
	2.2	What Medicare covers in a Skilled Nursing Facility	29
	2.3	Benefit period for a Skilled Nursing Facility	30
	3.	Home Health Care	33
	3.1	Home health-care benefits	34
	3.2	Additional home health-care benefits	35
	4.	Hospice Care	37
	4.1	What hospice care covers	37
	4.2	Other hospice issues	40

3 Part B: The Basics — 41

	1.	Part B Providers	41
	2.	Assignment	42
	3.	Filing Claims	46
	4.	Waiver of Liability: Advanced Beneficiary Notice	46

4 Part B: Details of Coverage — 49

	1.	The Most Commonly Covered Part B Services	49
	1.1	Doctors' services	50
	1.2	Radiology procedures	50
	1.3	Diagnostic tests	50
	1.4	Lab tests	51
	1.5	Hospital outpatient departments and clinics	51

1.6	Emergency rooms	51
1.7	Home health visits	51
1.8	Therapy	52
1.9	Ambulance	53
1.10	Pathology	53
1.11	Comprehensive Outpatient Rehabilitation Facilities (CORF)	53
1.12	Mental health services	54
1.13	Ambulatory surgical centers	55
2.	Information about Coverage for Other Services	55
2.1	Abdominal aortic screening	55
2.2	Abortion	56
2.3	Acupuncture	56
2.4	Alcoholism	56
2.5	Anesthesia	56
2.6	Artificial hearts	56
2.7	Blood	56
2.8	Bone mass measurement	56
2.9	Cardiac rehabilitation programs	57
2.10	Cardiovascular disease screening	57
2.11	Chemotherapy	57
2.12	Chiropractic	57
2.13	Clinical trials and research studies	57
2.14	Colorectal cancer screening	58
2.15	Community Mental Health Centers (CMHCs)	60
2.16	Cosmetic procedures	60
2.17	Dentistry	60
2.18	Diabetes screenings	60
2.19	Dialysis	62
2.20	Drug abuse and chemical dependency treatment	62
2.21	Drugs and biologicals	62
2.22	Eye coverage	63
2.23	Federally Qualified Health Clinics (FQHCs)	64
2.24	Flu vaccine	64
2.25	Foot care	64
2.26	Hearing aids and hearing exams	65
2.27	Hepatitis B vaccines	65
2.28	Inpatient ancillaries	65
2.29	Mammograms	65
2.30	Nutrition therapy	66

	2.31	Pap smear, pelvic exam, and breast exam	66
	2.32	Partial hospitalization	66
	2.33	Pathology	67
	2.34	Pneumonia or pneumococcal vaccine	67
	2.35	Portable X-rays and diagnostic X-rays	67
	2.36	Prostate cancer screening	67
	2.37	Radiation therapy	67
	2.38	Rural health clinic (RHC)	67
	2.39	Physician second and third opinions	68
	2.40	Smoking cessation counseling	68
	2.41	Telemedicine	68
	2.42	Transplants	68
	2.43	Transportation	68
	2.44	Vaccinations	69
	2.45	"Welcome to Medicare" Physical Exam	69

5 Part B: Durable Medical Equipment

5	**Part B: Durable Medical Equipment**	**71**
1.	Coverage of Durable Medical Equipment	72
2.	Equipment Must Be Supplied to Your Home	78
3.	Payment Methods for Durable Medical Equipment	78
	3.1 Low-cost or frequently purchased items	78
	3.2 Always rentals	79
	3.3 Capped rental items	79
4.	Extra Documentation on Durable Medical Equipment	80
5.	Advanced Determination of Medical Coverage	80
6.	If You Leave Original Medicare and Go to Medicare Advantage	81

6	**Part D: The Prescription Drug Benefit**	**83**
1.	The Part D Structure	83
	1.1 Deductible	84
	1.2 Basic benefit	84
	1.3 Coverage gap	85
	1.4 Catastrophic coverage	85
	1.5 Tiered payments	85
	1.6 Calculating your true out-of-pocket costs	85
2.	Enrollment Periods and Penalties	86
	2.1 Individual initial enrollment period	87
	2.2 Annual coordinated enrollment period	88
	2.3 Special enrollment periods	89
	2.4 Penalties	92
	2.5 Premium payments	93

	3.	Pharmacy Networks	93
	4.	Mail Order	94
	5.	Utilization Controls	94
	6.	Medication Therapy Management Programs	94
	7.	Part D: Details of Coverage	95
		7.1 How Part D works with Part A and Part B	95
		7.2 If you have Medicaid	96

7 Part D: Extra Help with Your Prescription Drug Benefit — 99

	1.	What Extra Help Covers	99
	2.	Automatic Qualification	101
	3.	Applying for Extra Help	101
	4.	Income and Resources for Extra Help Purposes	102
		4.1 Income	103
		4.2 Resources and assets	105
	5.	Special Family Situations	106
	6.	Special Circumstances in Qualifying for Extra Help	106
	7.	Premium Limits for Extra Help Beneficiaries	106
	8.	Changes and Redeterminations to Your Extra Help Status	108
		8.1 Subsidy changing events	109
		8.2 Redeterminations	109
		8.3 Extra Help notices	109
	9.	Appealing an Extra Help Decision	110

8 Part C: Medicare Advantage Plans and Enrollment Requirements — 113

	1.	Types of Medicare Advantage Plans	113
		1.1 Point-of-Service (POS) option	113
		1.2 Religious Fraternal Benefit plans	114
		1.3 Health Maintenance Organizations (HMO)	114
		1.4 Provider Sponsored Organizations (PSO)	114
		1.5 Preferred Provider Organizations (PPO)	114
		1.6 Special Needs Plans (SNP)	115
		1.7 Private Fee-for-Service (PFFS) plans	116
		1.8 Medical Savings Accounts (MSA)	117
		1.9 Cost plans	118
		1.10 Demonstration plans	118
		1.11 PACE plans	119
	2.	Enrolling in or Disenrolling from a Medicare Advantage Plan	119
		2.1 Initial coverage election period	119
		2.2 General enrollment period	120
		2.3 Open enrollment for newly eligible individuals	120

		2.4	Annual election period	121
		2.5	Open enrollment period	121
		2.6	Special enrollment periods	122
	3.		End-Stage Renal Disease and Medicare Advantage	127
	4.		The Grandfather Clause	128

9 Part C: Researching and Managing Medicare Advantage Plans — 129

	1.		Researching Plans	129
	2.		Common Marketing Scams	130
		2.1	Marketing restrictions on Medicare Advantage Plans	131
	3.		Important Plan Communications	132
		3.1	"Evidence of Coverage" booklet	132
		3.2	Annual Notice of Change	133
		3.3	Physician or health provider leaves the plan	134
	4.		Special Care Situations	134
		4.1	Emergency and urgently needed care	134
		4.2	Direct access to care situations	136
		4.3	Hospice care and Medicare Advantage	136
	5.		Your Special Rights and Protections in a Medicare Advantage Plan	136
		5.1	Change primary care physician	136
		5.2	Choose health-care providers	136
		5.3	Noninterference	137
		5.4	Compensation arrangements	137
		5.5	Second opinion	137
		5.6	Cultural competence	137
		5.7	Treatment plan	137
		5.8	Advance directives	138

10. Medigap: Medicare Supplement Insurance — 139

	1.		Medigap SELECT Policies	139
	2.		Medigap Structure and Benefits	140
		2.1	Basic benefits	140
		2.2	Part A inpatient deductible	142
		2.3	Skilled Nursing Facility	142
		2.4	Part B deductible	142
		2.5	Part B excess charges	142
		2.6	At-home recovery	142
		2.7	Foreign travel emergency	142
		2.8	Preventive care	143
		2.9	High deductible policies	143
		2.10	Catastrophic policies	143

3. Medigap Structure for Massachusetts, Minnesota, and Wisconsin   145
4. Variations in Policy Pricing   145
5. Information gathering   148
   5.1 Finding the policy that works for you   149
6. Discounts   150
7. Underwriting   150
   7.1 Preexisting conditions   150
8. Medigap Rights and Protections   151
   8.1 Your Medigap open enrollment period   151
   8.2 Your special guaranteed issue rights   151
   8.3 Disabled beneficiary's special suspension right   154
   8.4 Medicaid beneficiary's special suspension right   155
   8.5 Special Medigap consumer rights and protections   155
9. If You Kept a Medigap Policy with Drug Coverage   156
10. Contacting Companies   157
11. Major Medigap Changes in June, 2010   157
12. Medical Bill Tracking   157

11. Medicare and Private Health Insurance: Coordinating Your Benefits

       159
1. Coordination of Benefits   159
2. Employer and Union Group Health Insurance   160
   2.1 Retirement employer and union group health insurance   161
   2.2 Working employer and union group health insurance   162
   2.3 Consolidated Omnibus Budget Reconciliation Act (COBRA)   164
3. Workers' Compensation   168
   3.1 Conditional payment   168
   3.2 Set-aside arrangements   169
4. No-Fault and Liability Insurance   170

12. Coordinating Medicare with Government-Sponsored Health Programs

       171
1. Federal Black Lung Benefits Program   171
2. Veterans Benefits   172
   2.1 Coordination of Veterans Benefits with Part B and Part D   172
3. Civilian Health and Medical Program of the Department of Veterans Affairs (CHAMPVA)   173
   3.1 Coordination of CHAMPVA with Part A, Part B, and Part D   174
4. TRICARE For Life (TFL)   175
   4.1 Coordination of TRICARE For Life and Part A, Part B, and Part D   176
5. Federal Employee Health Benefits (FEHB)   177
   5.1 Federal Employee Health Benefits (FEHB) and Part B   178
   5.2 Federal Employee Health Benefits (FEHB) and Part D   179

	5.3	Primary payer rules	179
	5.4	Special rule for retirees who do not have Medicare	179
6.	Medicaid		180
	6.1	Medicaid and Part D	180

13. Specific Diseases and How Medicare Can Help

13.	**Specific Diseases and How Medicare Can Help**		181
1.	Diabetes		181
2.	Heart attack		182
3.	Alzheimer's Disease		183
4.	End-stage renal disease		184
	4.1	If you have Medicare and then get end-stage renal disease	184
	4.2	A special note on delaying your filing for Medicare	185
	4.3	End-stage renal disease beneficiaries and Medicare Advantage	186
	4.4	Termination of Medicare for end-stage renal disease beneficiaries	187
	4.5	Treatments and options	187
	4.6	End-stage renal disease networks	190

14. Medicare Appeals

14.	**Medicare Appeals**		193
1.	Some Helpful Guidelines for Medicare Appeals		193
	1.1	Amount in controversy	193
	1.2	Federal rules govern	194
	1.3	Forms	194
	1.4	Other entities appealing	194
	1.5	Representation	194
	1.6	Escalation	194
2.	Original Medicare Appeals		194
	2.1	Resubmittals	195
	2.2	Redeterminations	195
	2.3	Reconsiderations	195
	2.4	Administrative Law Judge hearings	196
	2.5	Medicare Appeals Council reviews	197
	2.6	US Federal District Court suits	197
	2.7	Your right to receive notice of and to appeal the termination of four specific services	197
	2.8	Appeals of local and national coverage determinations	199
3.	Medicare Managed Care Rights		200
	3.1	Right to a determination	201
	3.2	Your basic right to a decision on a claim and how to appeal it	204
	3.3	Right to file a grievance	205
	3.4	Right to express dissatisfaction about quality of care	206

4. Part D: Rights, Determinations, and Appeals 206
    4.1 Your special rights under Part D 207
    4.2 How to make a standard or normal time determination 208
    4.3 Expedited procedures 209
    4.4 Second level appeals: Reconsiderations 211
    4.5 Subsequent appeals 212

15. Your Rights as a Medicare Beneficiary: Know Them and Use Them!

      213
1. Entitlement and Enrollment Rights for Medicare Applicants and Beneficiaries 213
    1.1 Be protected against discrimination 213
    1.2 Receive services in a culturally competent way 214
    1.3 Get information from Medicare 214
    1.4 Participate in your health care decisions 214
    1.5 Advance notice for proposed medical care or treatment that is part of a research experiment 214
    1.6 Use advance directives 214
    1.7 File a complaint about the quality of your care 214
2. Your Beneficiary Rights in Original Medicare 216
    2.1 Free choice by patient and provider 216
    2.2 Obtain an itemized statement 216
3. Your Rights to Privacy Protections 216
4. Your Responsibilities 217

TABLES

1 Resource Limits for all Medicare Savings Programs 18
2 Monthly Income Limits for Qualified Disabled Working Individuals 18
3 Monthly Income Limits for Qualified Medicare Beneficiaries 18
4 Monthly Income Limits for Specified Low-income Medicare Beneficiaries 18
5 Monthly Income Limits for Qualified Individuals 18
6 For Single Persons and Married Couples Filing Jointly 19
7 For Married Persons Filing Separately 19
8 Part B Payments 44
9 Colorectal Screening Tests 59
10 Simplified Extra Help for 2009 (For lower 48 states only) 100
11 100 Percent of the Federal Poverty Limit (2009) 103
12 150 Percent of the Federal Poverty Limit (2009) 103
13 Extra Help Premium Benchmark Information 107
14 Open Enrollment Period Dos and Don'ts 122
15 Medigap Standard Policies 141
16 How Plans K and L Differ from the Standard Medigap Plans 144

NOTICE TO READERS

Laws are constantly changing. Every effort is made to keep this publication as current as possible. However, the author, the publisher, and the vendor of this book make no representations or warranties regarding the outcome or the use to which the information in this book is put and are not assuming any liability for any claims, losses, or damages arising out of the use of this book. The reader should not rely on the author or the publisher of this book for any professional advice. Please be sure that you have the most recent edition.

Note: The fees quoted in this book are correct at the date of publication. However, fees are subject to change without notice. For current fees, please check with the appropriate government office nearest you.

Prices, commissions, fees, and other costs mentioned in the text or shown in samples in this book probably do not reflect real costs where you live. Inflation and other factors, including geography, can cause the costs you might encounter to be much higher or even much lower than those we show. The dollar amounts shown are simply intended to be representative examples.

INTRODUCTION

As people age, many begin to prepare for their future health. As a result, entitlement to Medicare is not an issue for many when they retire. However, others do not realize how important it is to plan for retirement health concerns, even if they are in the midst of their retirement already or if they do not have any plans to retire.

This book is intended to provide you with the strategic basics you need to know to make wise choices with regard to your health plan. By the time you finish reading this book, you will know how to lower your costs while maximizing your Medicare benefits. This book also addresses other kinds of health insurance you may have, or may wish to get, in retirement.

People tend to think of the Medicare program as one for the elderly, but those on disability make up a considerable number of its beneficiaries. The Medicare program also serves people of all ages with end-stage renal disease.

Medicare also covers Social Security beneficiaries, but the list doesn't end there. Medicare covers those who are part of the Railroad Retirement System, a system which predates Social Security. Furthermore, those federal, state, and local government workers who are not covered by Social Security also pay into and receive Medicare. In this book, references to Social Security beneficiaries will include qualified government employees (working or retired) and those covered by the Railroad Retirement System.

People party neither to a pension system nor to Social Security coverage can also receive Medicare, but at a price.

If you are entitled to Medicare, you should think of it as your program — you are rightfully entitled to Medicare and its benefits by virtue of federal law and statute. You supported the system for all your working years, after all.

This book will let you know what your benefits are under the program and will inform you on how to use those benefits to your advantage. Your health is among your most valuable assets — this book will help you understand how to protect it to the best of your ability with Medicare.

Like many programs in America, Medicare is multigenerational. You were responsible during your working years for putting money into the system through wage deductions and self-employment taxes. Medicare used and continues to use that money to pay for its cost of operation. Now younger generations will have to do the same for you. Your children or kin will not, as individuals, have to be financially responsible for your health care, as they would have been before Medicare. This should give you an extra incentive to use the program wisely and to take responsibility for its proper use.

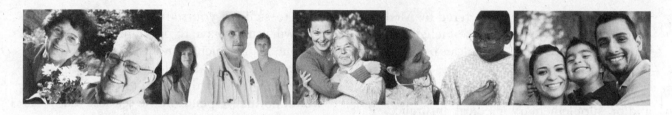

1

UNDERSTANDING THE BASICS OF ENROLLMENT IN AND ENTITLEMENT TO MEDICARE'S PROGRAMS

1. What is Medicare?

Essentially, Medicare is a social insurance system received by those aged 65 or over. It is designed to provide financial assistance for those at risk for requiring a moderate to high level of medical care. Medicare also covers disabled persons under the age of 65 and people of any age with end-stage renal disease. See Section 3. for details on eligibility.

There are many different programs within Medicare, within which there are subprograms to fit your precise needs. For now, let's introduce each of the main Medicare programs.

2. Medicare's Fundamental Programs

Let's begin by taking a quick look at Medicare's fundamental programs:

- Part A: Hospital insurance
- Part B: Medical insurance

- Part C: Medicare Advantage managed care and health plans
- Part D: Prescription drug insurance

These topics will be more detailed in the following chapters, but for now, let's begin with some of the basics.

Part A is also known as hospital insurance. It covers four kinds of care: hospital inpatient care, Skilled Nursing Facility inpatient care, home health care, and hospice care.

You can receive Part A if you are covered under Social Security, the Railroad Retirement System, or you are a qualified government employee, and if you are 65 or older, disabled, or have end-stage renal disease. Part A is free to receive provided that you have worked a minimum of 40 quarters (see section 4. for more on your options if not covered). If you begin to receive it when you are 65 or older, you'll have it for the rest of your life. Note that you usually have to receive Part A in order to be eligible for any of the other programs offered by Medicare. Section 4. discusses how those ineligible for receipt of Part A free of charge can buy their way into the program.

Part B is also known as medical insurance and/or supplementary medical insurance. Part B covers all sorts of physician, practitioner, and outpatient services.

Generally, you can receive Part B if you receive Part A and pay a monthly premium, which was $96.40 a month in 2009. If you are 65 years or older, you can continue to receive Part B for life, as long as you pay the premium. Because it is not free, some Medicare beneficiaries choose not to receive Part B; this will be discussed in depth in later chapters, as this is a critical decision. Note that it is possible for some people to receive Part B even if they don't qualify for Part A. However, not all recipients of Part A will visually be signed up for Part B automatically unless specified by the recipient otherwise.

Part A is known as Original Medicare, while Part B is called fee-for-service Medicare. Parts C and D are considered to be separate from Parts A and B; however, coverage for Parts C and D are contingent upon your coverage for Parts A and B, as we will see below.

Part C, known as Medicare Advantage, is slightly different than the other parts of Medicare because it is somewhat customizable. With Part C, you choose to receive your benefits through a separate health plan or managed care setting instead of through Original (or fee-for-service) Medicare. The benefit of this option is that when diverted through a separate health plan, your coverage could include such benefits as an annual cap on expenses which are not available under Original Medicare. Generally, you have to be entitled to both Part A and Part B to receive Part C. If you wish to receive your Medicare benefits in a Medicare Advantage health plan or managed care organization, you have to sign up yourself up with such a plan. You will usually have to pay a monthly premium to your plan, which is in addition to your Part B premium. Part C should not be taken lightly; the premium is worth paying to offset what you would normally spend on the services that Parts A and B do not cover.

Part D is also known as the prescription drug insurance, or the drug benefit. You are eligible to receive Part D if you have one or both of Part A or Part B, but you must sign up for it. You will typically pay a monthly premium, the amount of which varies widely.

While not all Medicare beneficiaries take advantage of Part D, it is an excellent insurance program which is helpful to those who require prescriptions for chronic conditions. You can receive Part D for life, as long as you continue to receive one or both of Part A or Part B and you pay the premiums. However, your particular plan may change from year to year. Furthermore, the particular drug plans you might join differ from one another depending on the state you live in.

Many Part C plans also have Part D coverage. If your Part C plan doesn't have drug coverage, you can sign up for an independent Part D drug plan.

When you become entitled to Medicare, you are enrolled automatically in Original Medicare, that is, Part A. With Original Medicare, you may go to any doctor or institution that provides Medicare-funded care; that is, you are able to direct your own care, choose your health-care providers, and decide when to get care.

If you don't have any health insurance apart from Medicare, you can buy a Medigap Policy, also known as Medicare Supplement Policy, if you cannot afford the substantial deductibles and coinsurance that Medicare requires you to pay. For more on Medigap, see Chapter 10.

This chapter discusses who is entitled to Part A and Part B. Note that you need to be receiving both Parts A and B in order to be eligible to take advantage of Part C, and you have to have at least one of Part A or Part B to be eligible for Part D. Chapters 2 through 9 will discuss these parts in more detail.

3. Entitlement

3.1 Entitlement based on a retirement account

Within three or four months of your 65th birthday, if you are signed up to receive your Social Security or Railroad Retirement benefits, you will automatically be enrolled in Part A and Part B. You will receive your red, white, and blue Medicare card.

If you are not signed up for monthly benefits through Social Security or the Railroad Retirement program, you need to apply for Medicare. This is true even if you won't actually be receiving a monthly benefit because you still work. This is because the Social Security Administration is the keeper of the records for all Medicare recipients (except for those in the Railroad Retirement System). If you are a federal, state, or local government worker and you have paid into Medicare but have not neccesarily paid into Social Security, you may get a government pension instead of Social Security benefits, and will have to sign up for Medicare manually.

Many people may want to apply for Medicare manually when they reach 65 because they are still working and want to take advantage of the Social Security provision that boosts their monthly benefit amount if they wait until past age 65 to retire. (These are called delayed retirement credits.) If this is what you want to do, you will have to call the Social Security Administration to file your application for delayed retirement credits. You should call four

months prior to your 65th birthday, as you may need to schedule an appointment at one of the local Social Security offices, which may entail a wait of several months depending on your area. Typically, you will have to prove your age and marital status to the Social Security Administration during this application process, although in most cases you can submit these documents by mail. These documents may include a birth certificate, marriage certificate, divorce decree, immigration papers, etc.

Note that you receive Medicare benefits by the calendar month, so if your 65th birthday is on July 27, you begin receiving Medicare on July 1.

There is a quirk in law for those few of you who were born on the first of a month. Medicare applies your birthday as though it fell on the day before it actually does, so you are considered 65 on the last day of the previous month. This means that you get Medicare for that whole month! For example, if your 65th birthday is on May 1, you will begin receiving Medicare on April 1.

Social Security uses the birthdate you wrote on your application for a social security number. If Social Security doesn't know your right age and birthdate, you will have to be proactive in making sure you get signed up. For example, if you deliberately used the wrong date trying to get a job or into the military when you were underage or you have subsequently learned your correct date of birth (this happens to immigrants born under a different calendar system), you will need to apply for Social Security and Medicare as you approach your correct age of 65.

On occasion, Social Security may have mixed up your earnings and coverage record with someone else's. In this case, it will review your records and straighten them out, but this takes some time. This is why it is important to apply a few months before you reach age 65. Social Security sends an annual letter to beneficiaries as they accumulate credits. This letter indicates what the projections are for each person's benefits. Hopefully, you have been verifying your information to be correct all along. If you haven't been receiving this information, you are probably not enrolled in the system; you'll need to contact Social Security and apply for benefits at least three months before your 65th birthday.

Other situations exist in which a family member of yours may want to apply for Medicare on your record before you become 65. For example, suppose your spouse is older than you and will reach age 65 before you do, but she is not covered by her own Social Security because she was a stay-at-home mom for her whole lifetime. She can apply and receive Medicare in this situation as soon as you are age 62, which is the earliest you can be entitled to retirement benefits, and she is 65, which is the earliest she can receive Medicare. If this is the case, she needs to apply for Medicare at least three months before she becomes 65. She will become entitled to Medicare as your spouse, but under her own Social Security number, even if you are still working. Social Security does this to encourage her to get Medicare as soon as she can without forcing you to file for your own monthly benefits, which would be established at a reduced rate as a result, even though you are working and would not yet receive payments. Your spouse won't be getting any cash benefits, at least until you file for Social Security. There is no loss or reduction to your cash benefits if your spouse applies for Medicare.

You should also be aware that there are other, rarer situations in which your dependents can file for Medicare on your Social Security earnings record without you being required to file your own Social Security benefits. Check with your local Social Security office if you are ever unsure about the coverage of dependents.

Children can also be entitled on their parents' accounts. If you have a disabled child, he or she might be eligible for Medicare on your retirement account. To be entitled, the child must qualify as a Social Security *disabled adult child.* (Sometimes the term *disabled child beneficiary* is used.) For the child to be eligible, five basic requirements must be met:

- The child must be at least 18 years of age.

- He or she has to be your child. This classification includes adopted children and, in some cases, stepchildren, grandchildren, or even step-grandchildren.

- The child has to be disabled according to the Social Security Administration's strict definition of disability.

- The disability (or accident) had to have manifested before he or she turned 22.

- The child cannot currently be married.

If you do have a disabled adult child, you need to keep this in mind: The child has to have been classified as a disabled adult child for 24 months before he or she becomes entitled to Medicare. Medicare entitlement must be applied for as early as possible (i.e., as you approach age 62 even if you won't actually retire and get payments) so he or she can serve his or her 24-month qualifying period in order to become entitled as soon as possible. Typically, the very earliest a disabled adult child can get Medicare is at age 20 (the minimum of age 18 plus the 24-month qualifying period).

This 24-month rule is waived if he or she has Lou Gehrig's disease, in which case his or her Medicare will begin as soon as he or she qualifies as a disabled adult child.

In summary, those applying through Medicare for their own coverage through the account of another person should —

- apply for Medicare as you, the official beneficiary approach 65 and your spouse is 62 or almost there; or

- as you, the parent, approach age 62 and your child is at least 18 or approaching that age.

Your entitlement to Medicare has nothing to do with whether or not you or your spouse are actually getting any Social Security retirement payments, but only whether you are 65 and could be entitled to Social Security on a spouse's account, which can be as early as the official beneficary's age is 62. Just a reminder; this also applies to those under the Railroad Retirement System and qualified government employees.

In some cases, a divorced spouse can get benefits on his or her ex-spouse's account. In those instances where one spouse is approaching 65 and the official beneficiary is 62 (or nearing 62), the first spouse, if he or she is not entitled to Medicare on his or her own account, should apply for Medicare as a divorced spouse. This application won't affect the ex at all; however, it is a fair and effective way to receive Medicare as well as possible monthly benefits.

Sometimes you can get Social Security cash benefits based on coverage you earned when you worked under the retirement system of another country. However, these will not be counted to see if you qualify for Medicare. If you do become entitled to Social Security retirement benefits based in part on another nation's retirement systems earnings, it is possible for you to get Social Security benefits, but not Medicare, even if you are 65.

3.2 Entitlement based on a survivor's account

Typically, survivor's benefits are for widows or widowers who qualify for benefits on a deceased spouse's Social Security account. They usually apply for these benefits as soon as they qualify (as early as age 60, if they are not working). When they turn 65, they are automatically entitled to Medicare.

In the case of disabled adult children, they can receive survivor's benefits on behalf of deceased parents after a 24-month qualifying period. These children must also meet the requirements discussed in section 3.1.

In rare cases, parents can be entitled to benefits on their deceased child's account. In order to do so, however, they have to meet a special dependency test. For example, suppose a hardworking immigrant brought his widowed (and penniless) mother to the United States to protect her from the political mayhem in their home country. As she is totally dependent on him for her support, if he were to die, she (who is older than 65) can become a Medicare beneficiary on his Social Security account. She may also be eligible for Social Security payments. As a noncitizen, however, she has to meet the necessary requirement of being lawfully present in this country for at least five years.

Besides disabled adult children, there is one special survivor category that can get Medicare before age 65: widows and widowers who are disabled but don't qualify for disability on their own accounts for whatever reason (for example, a stay-at-home parent who never worked). These people must meet the test for Social Security disability and be at least 50 years of age to become entitled to these special widow or widower disability benefits. Similar to disability beneficiaries (see section 3.3), they must be disabled for five full months before they become eligible for their disability entitlement. Similar to disabled adult children, they have a qualifying period of 24 months after they first become eligible to receive benefits. If you are in this category, it's important for you to apply for this benefit as early as possible, not only to get your monthly payments, but also to get your Medicare (you can get Medicare as early as age 52, or even age 50 if you have Lou Gehrig's disease). If you are eligible for Supplemental Security Income (SSI) or Supplemental State Payments based on a disability, you may count the months you were eligible for either of these toward both the 5-month waiting period and the 24-month qualifying period.

It's important to know that you don't necessarily have to be a disabled widow or widower beneficiary to get Medicare as such. Even if you become entitled as a widow or widower (which can happen as early as age 60), or if you are a "parent with children in your care" beneficiary at least 50 years of age, or even if you file for retirement on your own account as early as age 62, and you meet all the other requirements as a disabled widow or widower, you will be eligible for Medicare as soon as you meet the qualifying and waiting period requirements.

3.3 Entitlement based on a disability account

You should be aware that it takes a while for disability beneficiaries to get their Medicare. If you become disabled, your eligibility for payments does not begin until you have been disabled for five full calendar months. For example, if you were disabled in an accident on April 20, 2009, your eligibility for disability coverage doesn't begin until October 1, 2009. However, your Medicare coverage still doesn't begin until 24 months after you are eligible for payments. This means your Medicare won't be effective until October 1, 2011.

The five-month rule also applies to individuals getting disability on their own account and to disabled widows and widowers. Disabled adult children don't have to serve the 5-month waiting period, but they do have to wait the 24-month qualifying period for Medicare.

The one exception is if your disability is caused by Amyotrophic Lateral Sclerosis (ALS), often referred to as Lou Gehrig's disease. Your Medicare will begin as soon as your disability entitlement begins, which means you don't have to serve the 24-month qualifying period to get Medicare. This exception also applies to adult disabled children and disabled widows and widowers.

If you become a disability beneficiary on your own account, it may be possible for a spouse or former spouse to become entitled on your account when he or she reaches 65. Likewise, if a disabled adult child becomes entitled, he or she can get Medicare when he or she has served the 24-month qualifying period. Remember, in these situations, these people may be able to receive Medicare before you do.

Your entitlement to Medicare based on disability will end in two circumstances:

1. If your condition improves and Social Security ends your entitlement to disability payments, your Medicare ends the same month.

2. If you continue to be disabled yet engage in work to the extent that Social Security ends your benefit payments (called Qualified Disabled Working Individuals), your Medicare entitlement will continue for eight years and six months after you begin working. After that, you will have the option to buy Part A and Part B (and, if you purchase at least one of those parts, you can also apply for Part D) as long as Social Security continues to consider you disabled. For more information, read section 8.3 on Medicare Savings Programs — your state may help pay your premiums.

Sometimes it happens that even though you go off disability payments, you may become entitled to them again. If Social Security decides that your disability reoccurred within 60 months of your previous entitlement, you don't have to serve the five-month waiting period again; you become entitled to benefits right away. You don't have to serve the 24-month qualifying period for Medicare again, either — whatever months of previous entitlement you had can count toward that time. Also, regardless of the time span since your previous disability, if you become entitled due to the same condition for which you were previously entitled, you can count previous months toward this 24-month qualifying period, but, confusingly, these do not count toward the 5-month waiting period.

Remember that adult disabled children never have to serve the five-month waiting period. Note that disabled children and disabled widows and widowers have an 84-month span since their last entitlement (seven years), not just 60 months, to count previous months toward the 5-month requirement (this applies only to the widowed) and the 24-month qualifying period for Medicare.

If you are a disability beneficiary, you will be automatically switched to an aged beneficiary at age 65. The only difference the switch will make is that if you did not have Part B as part of your disability coverage, you will now be automatically enrolled in it. (You can refuse it, if you want to.) If you did have Part B, but for some reason you were paying a penalty on your Part B premium, that will be wiped out under aged beneficiary coverage and you will begin paying the standard premium amount. As long as you decide to keep your Part B enrollment, you also become eligible to buy a Medigap Policy of any type from any company that sells these in your area. (See Chapter 10 for more information about Medigap.)

If you become entitled to disability coverage on or after your 63rd birthday, you will automatically be enrolled in Part A and Part B as an aged beneficiary as of your 65th birthday. You don't have to wait the full 24 months. However, keep in mind that you will still have to consider whether to keep Part B, join Part C, or sign up for Part D.

3.4 Entitlement based on end-stage renal disease

Medicare is available to those who develop permanent kidney failure, usually called end-stage renal disease. This special provision was put in the law many years ago to enable affected people to undergo expensive kidney dialysis and transplant procedures without substantial financial hardship.

If you become eligible for Medicare this way, it helps pay for kidney treatment and for everything that Medicare covers; in other words, you get all the Medicare benefits. However, you can't join Part C of Medicare if you have end-stage renal disease. There are some exceptions to this rule; they are covered in Chapter 8.

If you are diagnosed with end-stage renal disease, you must file with Social Security or the Railroad Retirement Board and meet two specific requirements to get Medicare:

1. You have to be covered under Social Security, the Railroad Retirement Board, or as a qualified government employee. Keep in mind that you don't need as many quarters of coverage (or months, for Railroaders) to get this coverage requirement met as you do for retirement benefits. You can be the spouse or dependent child of someone who is covered. For example, if you are the spouse of one of the above-mentioned covered people, and you develop end-stage renal disease, you could become eligible for Medicare. Note that you do not have to be *dependent* on your covered spouse or

parent, and that the expansive definition of child (including adopted children and sometimes stepchildren, grandchildren, or step-grandchildren) is used here as with other entitlement approaches.

2. You have to get a kidney transplant or go on dialysis. The rules regarding your entitlement to Medicare are actually tied to which treatment you get. If you have never been a Medicare beneficiary because of end-stage renal disease and you go on dialysis, you become entitled to Medicare at the beginning of the fourth month of dialysis. In other words, if you begin dialysis on June 13, 2010, you become entitled to Medicare on September 1, 2010.

There is an exception to this: If when you go on dialysis you plan to go on self-dialysis, you participate in a Medicare approved self-dialysis training program, and you expect to complete this training, you will be covered by Medicare beginning with the first month in which you begin dialysis. This is done to encourage self-dialysis, which is less expensive for Medicare.

If you receive a kidney transplant, you are entitled to Medicare the month you receive the transplant, or the month you are admitted to a hospital to perform procedures leading to one, provided that the actual transplant takes place in the following two months. Note that Medicare approves only certain hospitals to do kidney transplants, and your hospital has to be one of the approved for your coverage to kick in.

However, if you have previously been a Medicare beneficiary because of end-stage renal disease and you begin dialysis, you are entitled to Medicare beginning on the month you begin dialysis. You will have to file a new application with Social Security or the Railroad Retirement Board for this new entitlement.

This benefit is unique in Medicare because if a transplant is covered, it will pay the costs of the live kidney donor's medical expenses for donating the kidney (and costs for complications, if any, from the donation). The donor does not get Medicare, but his or her expenses related to the procedure are billed to and covered by Medicare.

Unlike entitlement to Medicare because of a retirement, as a survivor, or with a disability benefit, only the person with kidney disease gets Medicare. No one else in the family receives coverage, even if the person receives it on his or her spouse's or parent's account.

Similar to disability Medicare, it is possible that your Medicare coverage can end because of a positive change in your medical condition — in this case, because your kidney condition improves. If you no longer need dialysis, your entitlement to Medicare will end 12 months after the month you did not require dialysis. For example, you last had dialysis on April 21, 2010, your entitlement to Medicare will end April 1, 2011.

It is more likely your entitlement will end because of a successful transplant. In this case, Medicare will end with the 36th month after your kidney transplant. For instance, you had a transplant on September 12, 2010, your Medicare entitlement will end October 1, 2013.

There is some good news and bad news for those who already have Medicare and then get end-stage renal disease. When you are diagnosed and begin treatment, if you do not have Part B, you will be given the opportunity to sign up for it. If you do have Part B and you are paying a penalty premium, the penalty will be dropped. However, as with those who are actually entitled to Medicare because of this disease, you cannot join a Medicare Advantage managed care or health plan.

3.5 Retroactive Part A entitlement

You should be aware that it is possible to get entitled to Part A retroactively. The Social Security Administration has a whole set of rules about whether or not, when you file for benefits, your application can be effective for months before it is actually filed. The rules are complicated and depend on many factors.

In disability cases, retroactivity can sometimes be established for up to 12 months; in retirement and survivors' cases, sometimes for up to 6 months. Even within these rules, there are exceptions that allow certain applications to be retroactive solely for entitlement to Part A. For example, disabled widows filing for benefits may be allowed 12 months of retroactivity, which permits them to count these months toward their 24-month waiting period. Those filing for entitlement based on end-stage renal disease can always have their entitlement to Medicare established up to 12 months before their month of filing if they meet all other requirements in those months. The best advice is to contact Social Security and file as early as possible. If appropriate, you can always ask about retroactivity.

You should know that Part B and Part D cannot usually be made retroactive for months before you file. The exception to this is that those becoming entitled to Part A as an end-stage renal disease beneficiary can also elect Part B retroactively for up to 12 months. They would, however, be responsible for the Part B premiums for the months elected.

4. Buying into Medicare: Premium Part A

This section applies to you only if you don't have free Part A (that is, if you haven't worked a minimum of 40 quarters) and you are a US citizen age 65 or older; an alien lawfully admitted and present in this county (i.e., you have your I-155 or "green card") for at least five years and are 65 or older; or a disability beneficiary going off Medicare after eight-and-a-half years of substantial gainful employment while still medically disabled.

You may purchase Medicare Part A by paying a premium for it. The premium is calculated depending on whether you have a minimum amount of Social Security or Railroad coverage from work or self-employment. If you have none or less than 30 quarters of coverage, you pay the standard premium; and if you have at least 30 quarters, you pay the reduced premium. In 2010 these amounts are the following:

- Standard Part A Monthly Premium: $461
- Reduced Part A Monthly Premium: $254

While these are steep prices, Part A is possibly the least expensive insurance you can get for what it covers. If you buy Part A, and only if you do, you may also purchase Part B and/or Part D. If you buy both Part A and Part B, you can join a Part C Medicare Advantage managed care or health plan. You should seriously consider Part A either as an ongoing option or for temporary entitlement until you can be covered by some other means. For example, it was discussed earlier where a wife is not covered by her own Social Security and she would apply for Medicare when her husband becomes or is approaching 62. What if the husband isn't yet 62 and his wife could not get Medicare even though she is 65? She may want to consider purchasing Part A until her husband reaches age 62.

A spouse, widower, or divorced spouse can, under most circumstances, use the quarters of coverage of his or her current spouse, deceased spouse, or former spouse to qualify for the reduced premium. The age of either person does not matter. This option will automatically be considered when you apply, and may actually make the purchase of Part A affordable for you.

You should consider the purchase option when you first become 65. The reason is because you can make the decision to purchase Part A only during an enrollment period. (For more information on enrollment periods, see section 5.) Basically the enrollment period is the month you become 65 and the three months before and after this (a period of seven months altogether) and the first three months of every calendar year. The insurance will not always go into effect immediately; for example, if you enroll during a calendar-year enrollment period, it will not begin until July 1 of that year. Purchasing Plan A will give you initial coverage while you wait for your paid coverage to kick in.

Another reason you should consider taking the purchase option is that the amount of the premium will go up by 10 percent if you could have had, but did not have, Part A for at least 12 months. For instance, suppose you became 65 on June 12, 2009, and you decided, in the next calendar-year enrollment period (starting in February of 2009), to purchase it. Your premium would be $507.10 (or $461 plus 10 percent) and your Medicare Part A won't kick in until July 1, 2010. The penalty for the reduced Part A premium is $279.40 in 2009. Note that unlike Part B or Part D, in Part A you either get a flat-rate penalty or you don't — the amount does not go up if you delay even longer.

However, there is some good news. If you are paying a penalty premium for your Part A, it will eventually go back down to the standard rate. The rule here is that you will have to pay your penalty premium for twice the amount of time that you could have had Part A but didn't, and then the premium will revert to the standard rate. For example, you will have to pay the penalty premium for July 2010 to June of 2012 (two years) because you were one year late in becoming entitled. The government will keep track of this and change your premium automatically.

You should keep another strategy in mind. You should consider going to work or becoming self-employed to build up your Social Security quarters of coverage so you can qualify for the reduced premium. Note that it is $207 a month less than the standard in 2010. That's a lot of money each month. If you have 22 quarters, and you work two years to get 8 more, you'll have a total of 30 quarters, and you qualify for the reduced premium. If you continue to earn quarters and you accumulate a total of 40, as soon as you do, you may qualify for full Social Security entitlement, in which case you will get your Part A for free.

You will be terminated from Part A coverage if you don't pay your premium. (Asking to be terminated is probably not a good option, as you will have to pay back any Part A claims payments made on your behalf.) However, note that you can rejoin only during an enrollment period. If you allow your plan to expire, your premiums will almost certainly go up when you reapply. Remember, if you are younger than 65, you can't get Part B without having Part A, so if your Part A terminates, you will also be dropped from Part B if you have it. You can't have Part D without one of Part A or Part B, so you will also be dropped from Part D if you let Part A be terminated.

If you have limited income and resources, read section 8.3 about Medicare Savings Programs. If you meet the requirements as a Qualified Disabled Working Individual or a Qualified

Medicare Beneficiary, your state may pay your Part A premium.

There also exists a special provision for certain individuals to have their premium reduced to zero. If you are married to, or are widowed by a former state, county, or local government employee (or are one yourself), you are eligible for this provision. Certain dependents who have paid their Part A premiums for 84 months (seven years) can have their premium reduced to zero. They must meet several other requirements. As you approach seven years of payment, you may receive a form confirming your eligibility for premium-free benefits. If you don't receive this form, you should request one.

5. Enrollment Periods

Once you are receiving Part A of Medicare, you have to think about whether or not to enroll in Part B. It used to be that when you were automatically signed up at age 65 for Part A, it was up to you to sign up to Part B. However, since just about everybody did sign up, now the government presumes you want Part B — it is now up to you to take action if you *don't* want it.

If you reach age 65 and don't receive Part A, you can sign up for Part B. The rule is that if you are 65 or older, a resident of the US, and a US citizen (or a lawfully admitted alien who has lived in the US continuously for five full years), you can buy Part B without having to buy Part A. You may also get a chance to enroll in Part D, effective the date your Part B coverage starts. Keep in mind that this only applies if you are over 65; if you are younger than 65, you must receive Part A in order to receive Part B.

If you don't have any other health insurance, it is strongly advised that you receive Part B. Some health insurance plans insist that you join Part B in order to be eligible for health insurance, as is the case with TRICARE For Life.

Some employers or unions will pay your Part B premium; for example, the United Mine Workers (UMW) union pays the Part B premium for its retired members.

Medicare sets the Part B premium so that you pay 25 percent of the costs of the Part B medical insurance program, with the Medicare Trust Fund paying the other 75 percent. In 2010, the premium is $110.40 a month. The premium has been rising sharply in the last few years.

You can't simply begin receiving Part B whenever you decide you want it. As with most health insurance programs, there is an *enrollment period* to sign up for Part B. While you are automatically signed up for Part B when you begin receiving Part A at age 65, acquire a disability, or have end-stage renal disease, and you drop Part B and then want it later, you usually have only the first three months of a calendar year to sign up for it. In such circumstances, it doesn't go into effect until July 1 of that year.

If you choose not to enroll in Part B at your first opportunity, or if you drop it and sign up for it again at a later date, you will pay an increased premium. Specifically, the increase is 10 percent for each 12 months you could have been enrolled but were not. For example, you may decide at age 65 that you'll wait until you are 70 to get Part B, and you enroll then (presuming all this works out with the enrollment periods); you could have had it for 5 years. Your premium penalty will be 50 percent, which means you'll pay $165.70 a month instead of the original $110.50.

The penalty is refigured every year when the Part B premium goes up by multiplying the new, full premium amount by your applicable percentage, not just by adding your original penalty amount to the new premium amount. Seeing that the premium usually goes up steeply, the penalties get worse every year. Note that this penalty never expires, except in the unusual cases discussed in section 7.7.

You are better off with the extra coverage, which you can always drop rather than being stuck with unanticipated medical bills. It is important for you to plan ahead when you are enrolling in Medicare to get your preventative health exams started; these are always covered by Part B. See the "Welcome to Medicare" Physical Exam (section **2.45** in Chapter 4) to get going on this.

If you decide that you want to end your Part B enrollment, call Social Security Administration; they will send you a form to sign, and will probably try to set up an interview with you to make sure you understand what you are doing. If you do file the form or a written request to terminate, your Part B will end on the last day of the following month. You will still be responsible for your premiums due through that month.

There are several times you can enroll for Part B:

- when you are first eligible at age 65,
- when your individual enrollment period occurs. You have a specific period in which you can enroll which provides entitlement to Part B. If you sign up during this period, you will not be subject to any premium penalty,
- during a general enrollment period which occurs every year, or
- during a special enrollment period.

5.1 Individual enrollment periods

For those turning 65, the individual enrollment period is typically the month you turn 65, the three prior months, and the three following months.

The rules call for you to sign up for Part B during the three months prior to your 65th birthday to receive coverage on the month you turn 65 — your earliest opportunity to receive coverage. If you sign up the month you become 65, you begin receiving coverage the following month. If you sign up two months after you turn 65, your coverage begins after you sign up. If you sign up either of the two remaining months, your coverage begins three months after you sign up.

For alien residents, you will need to fit the requirements of being both 65 and having resided lawfully in the US for five full years (i.e., 60 full calendar months). For example, if you are already 65 and you arrived here on April 23, 2005, your 60th month will be April, 2010, and your eligibility will begin in May, 2010 (the month you met both requirements) with your initial enrollment period beginning on February 1, 2010.

5.2 General enrollment periods

If you opt out of Medicare Part B during your initial enrollment period, you have another chance to enroll each and every calendar year and to sign up during the general enrollment period from January 1 through March 31. Your coverage begins the following July 1. Your monthly premium increases 10 percent for each full 12 months you were eligible, but did not enroll in, Medicare Part B.

If you do not receive Part A, you meet the requirements to sign up for Part B, and you enroll during a general enrollment period, you also get a special enrollment period to sign up for Part D. This period begins April 1 and goes through June 30 (i.e., it immediately follows the Part B general enrollment period). If you sign up for Part D during this period, your coverage will begin July 1, which is when your Part B coverage takes effect. The following sections discuss special enrollment periods in more detail.

5.3 Employer and union group health special enrollment period

One of the most important special enrollment periods comes if you are 65 or older when your Employer Group Health Plan (EGHP) ends. If you have EGHP insurance through the employment of you or your spouse, and you are 65 or older, you can enroll in Part B at any time. If you lose this coverage (e.g., when you retire, your employment ends, or your company terminates health benefits), or you decide to quit the plan, you get a special enrollment period: You may enroll on the month your coverage ends, the month you are no longer employed, or during any of the following eight months in either of these circumstances.

If you take advantage of this special enrollment period, you will not pay any penalty on your Part B premium, even if you had previously disconnected Part B and you previously had to pay a premium penalty for whatever reason.

If you sign up on the month your coverage ends, you may choose to begin your Part B that month or during any of the next three months. If you sign up during any of the remaining eight months of your special enrollment period, Part B will automatically begin the following month.

Remember, you can sign up for Part B anytime that you have coverage. You can start Part B within the month that you sign up or any of the following three months.

Warning: In any of these situations, you need to know that you automatically start your Medigap open enrollment period when you enroll for Part B. If you are planning to get Medigap insurance, you need to get it at this time. This will be your only opportunity for a Medigap open enrollment period. Also note that if you previously had Part B and dropped it after age 65, and you began coverage under an EGHP at the later date, you do not get another Medigap open enrollment period.

There is another tricky issue to be aware of: If you are age 65 or older and you get your EGHP in a company with fewer than 20 employees, you should talk to your employee health benefits administrator before making a decision not to receive Medicare Part B. This is because your health insurance will be secondary to Medicare. In other words, Medicare will pay first and then your company plan will pay on the remaining amount. If you don't have Part B, your company may pay nothing because Medicare didn't pay its share. Even though you will keep your EGHP insurance, you also need to sign up for Part B. Be sure to talk to your company's employee health benefits administrator to understand exactly how the company's plan works.

Also, if you have a disability, and you become entitled to Medicare, your EGHP insurance will be the primary payer if your company (or the company of your spouse) has 100 or more employees. Again, Part B will be of limited value to you. However, if you lose this coverage, you get a special enrollment period and no penalty if you sign up in that period. If the company has fewer than 100 employees, you will want Part B. Again, be sure to talk to your company's employee health benefits administrator to understand exactly how the company's plan works.

5.4 Foreign situations

A special enrollment period also exists if you are a US citizen living abroad, you are age 65 or older, you are *not* eligible for Social Security or Railroad benefits, not eligible for Part A, and you return to the US to establish residence. You are allowed a special initial enrollment period, with the enrollment period being the month you return to the US and the three previous and three subsequent months. This enrollment period exists because, if you don't get Social Security or Railroad benefits, you can't get Part B if you don't reside in the US. Also note that you don't have to pay any penalty on your Part B premium if you use this special enrollment period.

5.5 International volunteers

A fairly recent change in the law allows Medicare beneficiaries to postpone or suspend their Part B enrollment when they perform volunteer services abroad for, or under the sponsorship of, an organization that the Internal Revenue Service (IRS) recognizes as tax exempt. The organization's volunteer service must be at least 12 consecutive months long, and the volunteer must be covered by health insurance while performing this volunteer service. This coverage does not necessarily have to be supplied by the volunteer organization, although this is typically the case.

If you are in this situation, when the volunteer service has ended and you return to the US, you get a six-month special enrollment period to enroll or re-enroll in Part B. Part B will go into effect the month after you request enrollment. The months that you were volunteering will *not* count toward any premium penalty.

This special enrollment period, in effect, allows beneficiaries who meet its requirements to safely terminate their Part B enrollment when they go abroad as a volunteer, and to get it back when they return. Medicare recognizes that Part B won't cover anything while you are in a foreign land, so there is no sense paying the premiums during that time. Also, if you happen to be one of the few beneficiaries who have Premium Part A, you may be able to suspend it under this provision. Check with Social Security or your international volunteer organization.

6. How Part B Coordinates with Your Other Health Insurance

The most difficult factor for you to consider in deciding whether or not to enroll in Part B comes if you have other health insurance. You have to figure out how your other health insurance works with Medicare, and then decide whether to keep it and not take Part B, take Part B and drop your other insurance, or stay with your insurance and get Part B. The answers here are not always easy because you have to understand how your insurance works with Medicare Part B. Figuring out what your plan pays for and what Medicare does and how they work together is similar to solving a two-part equation.

For example, if you are a retired federal employee, you carried health insurance for the five years before you retired, and you paid your monthly premiums, you can stay in the federal employee health program in retirement. You get Medicare Part A because you have paid into it through the years as a qualified government employee, so you need to decide whether to take Part B or not.

The first question you have to consider is whether your retirement medical insurance has you in managed care or fee-for-service. Generally, if you are in managed care, as long as you stay with your plan's provider network and its preapproval and other rules, you'll mostly be charged co-payments and maybe some other costs. If you're happy with your health maintenance organization (HMO), you probably don't need Part B.

Conversely, if you are in fee-for-service, you need to consider how your retirement medical plan coordinates with Part B; that is, you need to figure out what Medicare will pay along with what your retirement medical insurance pays. It's hard enough understanding one system let alone two, but the way you do this is to carefully review your retirement medical insurance brochure's explanation of how it coordinates with Part B. You can also talk to a retirement specialist in your human relations department at your work, or talk to some of your former coworkers who have retired. The best general advice is that unless your fee-for-service retirement medical insurance is quite generous, you should take Part B.

For more information about coordinating your benefits, see Chapters 11 and 12.

7. Noncoverage outside the US

This section is here for two reasons. The first reason is make sure that before you receive Part B, you understand that Medicare doesn't cover care you receive outside the US. You don't want to be paying Part B premiums if you don't need to, for example, if you plan to live abroad after you retire. The second reason is to briefly discuss what little it does cover in foreign situations.

This did not used to seem to be an important issue, but recent studies have shown that there are millions of Americans living permanently abroad. Another trend has grown too: that of "medical tourism." This occurs when patients go to foreign counties to receive medical treatment, both elective and nonelective. These trips may involve going across the Mexican or Canadian border for a dental procedure, or a halfway around the world to New Delhi for a heart operation. Something else to consider is the use of foreign Internet pharmacies and other sources to buy prescription drugs.

Medicare has not changed with the times and does not pay for health care outside the US, although there are a few exceptions. (Note that Puerto Rico, the US Virgin Islands, and the

Pacific territories of Guam, American Samoa, and the Northern Mariana Islands are part of the US. Medicare covers your care in those places.)

The first exception to the no foreign coverage rule occurs if you are traveling without unreasonable delay, between Alaska and the "lower 48." For instance, if you are travelling the most direct route between Alaska and Washington state and a medical emergency occurs (e.g., heart attack or vehicle accident), and the nearest hospital is Canadian, you are covered for Canadian treatment. Note, however, that it *must* be in an emergency situation.

The second exception, similarly, dictates that if you are in the US when a medical emergency occurs (e.g., sudden illness or injury), and there is a foreign hospital closer to you than the nearest US hospital, Medicare will cover you.

The third exception dictates that if you live in the US, but there is a foreign hospital closer to your home than the nearest US hospital that can treat your medical condition, you are covered at the foreign hospital. This differs from the second exception in that there is no requirement that you must be in an emergency situation, but the bearing is on your home's location rather than your location.

With regard to these exceptional circumstances, Medicare will cover you only if you are admitted to a (foreign) hospital as an inpatient. It will cover only your inpatient hospital care, doctors' services to you as an inpatient, and the ambulance trip to the hospital if you are admitted as an inpatient. In other words, you remain uncovered for outpatient care even given extenuating circumstances.

The fourth exception dictates that, in limited circumstances, Medicare will cover care provided by a ship's doctor on a cruise ship if it is in or near a US port. The rules are a little convoluted, so if you receive care in such a situation and you are billed, call Medicare to ask if you should submit a claim.

There are two other exceptions: First, some Medicare Advantage managed care or health plans (for instance, Part C) will cover much more care in a foreign locale than will Original Medicare. If you travel abroad extensively, you may wish to look for such a plan and sign up for it. Second, many Medigap insurance policies have a foreign travel provision; this is discussed further in Chapter 10. However, neither of these exceptions are relevant to Part B coverage.

You can see why most people who live abroad don't take Part B. Unless you are in a situation in which you have to have Part B (e.g., you have health insurance that requires you to get Part B), it wouldn't make sense to get it. Or unless you are thinking of returning to the US in the near future, or if you live close by and you plan to get your medical care in the US.

8. Getting Help Paying Your Part B Premium

8.1 The Social Security savings clause

The Social Security savings clause provides relief from excessive increases in the Part B premium when compared to increases in the Social Security benefit. It doesn't actually pay for your premium, but it takes measures to keep it in check. Because annual cost-of-living increases for Social Security beneficiaries are based on the general inflation rate while the increases in Part B premiums are based on increases in Medicare spending, Part B premiums usually go up much faster than Social Security benefits. The law provides that when the increase in value of your Part B premium exceeds the increase in value of your Social Security payment, the amount you receive from Social Security payments will not go down — it will stay the same. This is arranged by reducing your Part B premium so that your cash benefit payment does not change. This clause typically applies to those who are getting fairly modest monthly benefits.

The clause does not apply if your total Social Security payment is less than the total Part B premium. This usually would occur because your Social Security was subject to the government pension offset rules.

8.2 Medicaid

People on Medicaid as well as Medicare, often known as *dual eligibles*, generally have their Medicare Part B premium paid by their state's Medicaid program. If you, or someone you know, are on Medicaid, make sure that Medicaid is paying your Part B premium.

8.3 Medicare Savings Program

The Medicare Savings Program is an important state program that helps certain people with low income and few resources pay their Medicare premiums, and sometimes their deductibles and coinsurance. These people are variously called Qualified Disabled Working Individuals, Qualified Medicare Beneficiaries, Specified Low-Income Medicare Beneficiaries, and Qualified Individuals.

Briefly put, you have to meet both an income test and a resources test to qualify for a savings program. If your monthly income is low (see Tables 1–7 for the monthly limits; these are based on the Federal Poverty levels and change every year) and your resources are worth less than $4,000 for an individual and $6,000 for a married couple, you may qualify. Resources do not include your home, the land it's on, your car, or your personal effects, but include cash and savings bonds.

Some states have their own programs similar to the Medicare Savings Program, but these state programs have higher limits. If you apply for the Medicare Savings Program, the states that have their own programs will automatically consider you for their programs. The key here is that resources and income are counted differently in each state, so if you are anywhere near the limits shown in the tables below, apply. If your state has a program, you will be considered.

Critically important in thinking of applying for these savings programs is that what qualifies as *income* and *resources* tends to be a very complicated matter. There are many exclusions, disregards, and rules when there are more than two people in the household with regard to what counts as income. State rules vary from place to place, but each state also has a different interpretation of the federal rules.

Talk to your state Medicaid people or your State Health Insurance Assistance Program (SHIP) counselors for more information. Remember that many states have programs that expand on these.

For all of these programs you must have Medicare Part A and meet the resource limits in Table 1.

8.3a Qualified Disabled Working Individuals

If you are entitled to Social Security disability but went back to work in spite of your disability and intend to keep working for eight-and-a-half years, you can qualify for this program if your resources and income are both less than shown in Table 2. Note that the income limits for this program are comparatively generous, which is an attempt to keep you working. This program will pay your Part A premium only.

8.3b Qualified Medicare Beneficiaries

If you meet the income limits in Table 3, you will not only get your premiums for both Part A and Part B paid, but you will also have your Part A and Part B deductibles paid, and your Part B coinsurance amounts as well (although there is some variation between states). This is similar to having a Medigap policy coupled with paid premiums.

8.3c Specified Low-Income Medicare Beneficiaries

If you don't meet the income limits in Table 3 but you do meet the higher limits of Table 4, your state will pay your Part B premium. That's close to $100 per month for one person!

8.3d Qualified Individuals

If you don't meet the income limits in Tables 1 through 4 but you do meet the limits in Table 5, your state will pay your Part B premium. That's close to $100 per month per person!

8.4 Payment by employer, union, or other organization

There are employers and unions that pay the Part B premium for members who are on Medicare, and they pay the government directly. Be sure to ask your current or former employer, union, or civic organization if they do this. Note that they can't do this if you are getting Social Security, are part of the Railroad Retirement program, or are receiving a federal pension.

8.5 Reimbursement programs

Many retirement programs help their beneficiaries with their Part B premiums, reimbursing them for all or part of it. The typical reimbursement is 50 percent, but some retirement programs pay 100 percent. Note that most of these programs will reimburse you only the standard premium, not any additional penalty you may have. While your premium is deducted from your government retirement check, you are eventually reimbursed.

TABLE 1
RESOURCE LIMITS FOR ALL MEDICARE SAVINGS PROGRAMS

48 states + Washington, DC		Alaska		Hawaii	
Single	Couple	Single	Couple	Single	Couple
$4,000	$6,000	$4,000	$6,000	$4,000	$6,000

TABLE 2
MONTHLY INCOME LIMITS FOR QUALIFIED DISABLED WORKING INDIVIDUALS

48 states + Washington, DC		Alaska		Hawaii	
Single	Couple	Single	Couple	Single	Couple
$1,805	$2,428	$2,255	$3,035	$2,077	$2,793

TABLE 3
MONTHLY INCOME LIMITS FOR QUALIFIED MEDICARE BENEFICIARIES

48 states + Washington, DC		Alaska		Hawaii	
Single	Couple	Single	Couple	Single	Couple
$903	$1,214	$1,128	$1,518	$1,038	$1,397

TABLE 4
MONTHLY INCOME LIMITS FOR SPECIFIED LOW-INCOME MEDICARE BENEFICIARIES

48 states + Washington, DC		Alaska		Hawaii	
Single	Couple	Single	Couple	Single	Couple
$1,083	$1,457	$1,353	$1,821	$1,246	$1,676

TABLE 5
MONTHLY INCOME LIMITS FOR QUALIFIED INDIVIDUALS

48 states + Washington, DC		Alaska		Hawaii	
Single	Couple	Single	Couple	Single	Couple
$1,218	$1,639	$1,522	$2,049	$1,402	$1,886

8.6 Your Medicare Advantage Part C health plan

Some Medicare Advantage managed care or health plans (i.e., Part C plans) will pay part of your Part B premium if you enroll with them. While this happens only in limited parts of the US, you should consider taking advantage of this competition.

9. Part B: High-Income Premium Surcharges

This section will help you calculate the amount of your surcharge. The following tables show what one person's monthly premium amount is in 2010.

Table 6 shows, in the first row, that if you have an annual income less than $85,001 (if single) or less than $171,000 (if a couple filing jointly), you will not pay a surcharge for Part B coverage. The next rows show the percent of the total cost of Part B you will pay, the actual monthly premium you will have to pay, and how much more a month this premium is over and above the standard $110.50 a month for each respective income range. Table 7 shows similar information for married people who file separately.

If you are subject to a premium surcharge, it is applied to your Part B premium by adding it to the standard amount. However, if you are paying a penalty on your Part B premium because you did not enroll as soon as you could

TABLE 6
FOR SINGLE PERSONS AND MARRIED COUPLES FILING JOINTLY

Individual's Income Range	Couple's Income Range	Percent of Cost You Pay	Your Premium in 2010	Surcharge You Pay in 2010
Less than $85,001	Less than $171,000	25%	$110.50	$0.00
$85,001 – $107,000	$171,001 – $214,000	35%	$154.70	$44.20
$107,001 – $160,000	$214,001 – $320,000	50%	$221.00	$110.50
$160,001 – $214,000	$320,001 – $428,000	65%	$287.30	$176.80
More than $214,001	More than $428,001	80%	$353.60	$243.00

TABLE 7
FOR MARRIED PERSONS FILING SEPARATELY

Individual's Income Range	Percent of Cost You Pay	Your Premium in 2010	Surcharge You Pay in 2010
Less than $85,001	25%	$96.40	$0.00
$85,001 – $129,000	65%	$287.30	$176.80
More than $129,001	80%	$353.60	$243.10

(recall that this is 10 percent for each 12 month period that you could have been signed up for Part B but you weren't), the premium surcharge is not increased by your penalty percentage; it remains a set figure. The penalty percentage is applied only to the standard, base premium, and not to the adjustment. The following example will help you calculate this:

- Standard Part B premium for 2010: $110.50

- You are subject to a 10 percent late filing penalty: $11

- Standard plus late enrollment penalty: $121.50

- Your high-income premium surcharge: $44.20

- Your total Part B monthly premium: $165.70

9.1 Modified Adjusted Gross Income (MAGI)

You may get a letter from the Social Security Administration telling you that you will be assessed a higher premium for your Medicare Part B because of your income. Note that this letter is a predetermination letter, which basically informs you of what is going on, and gives you the opportunity to disagree. A few weeks after you receive this predetermination letter, you will also get a formal determination letter that will tell you all of this again, and it will give you your formal appeal rights to the decision.

If you are already on Medicare and then become subject to the premium surcharge, you will learn this when you get your annual letter from Social Security telling you how much your increase in Social Security will be the next year due to the rise in cost of living. These letters are usually sent out in November. (Note: Railroad Retirement Board and federal civil service annuitants will get a letter from the Social Security Administration, and also a letter from their respective payers.)

More specifically, these letters will explain that MAGI means your Modified Adjusted Gross Income. Your adjusted gross income is taken from line 37 of your tax return, Form 1040. For Part B premium purposes, this sum is modified by adding to it the amount on line 8b of the same form, which is any tax-exempt interest you earned, such as interest from tax-exempt state and municipal bonds.

On a Form 1040A, the adjustable gross income is on line 21 and the tax-exempt income is on line 8b; and on the Form 1040EZ, your adjustable gross income is on line 4. You can't use Form 1040EZ if you are 65 or older, but remember Social Security looks at your return from two or three years back, and both disabled and end-stage renal disease beneficiaries are subject to this premium surcharge.

Unfortunately for you, the MAGI letters will probably be accurate, and, unless one of the exceptions detailed in section 9.2 applies to you, you'll probably have to pay the higher premium.

9.2 Requesting a change in premium surcharge

It may be that something has happened that will help you lower or eliminate your premium surcharge. For instance, suppose the Social Security Administration used the wrong year to determine your income-related premium surcharge. The MAGI letter won't explain this well, but Social Security generally uses your tax return from the year prior to when you get the decision about what you will be paying in the next calendar year. If Social Security is figuring out what your premium should be in 2010, it does this in 2009, and it uses your 2008 income tax return. This is because at the time it makes its determination, this prior year is usually the latest return it has available from the Internal Revenue Service (IRS).

It may also be that the Social Security Administration used a return from an earlier year. For example, say it did not have your 2008 return — it used instead your 2007 return to calculate your 2010 premium surcharge. This can happen as a result of delays. If this occurs and if your correct year's return (i.e., 2008) information would lower or eliminate your premium surcharge, contact the Social Security Administration. Take everything into account when discerning whether you are entitled to a rebate: Perhaps your income went down, or you used a different filing status. Be prepared to submit the tax return that the Social Security Administration doesn't have.

In a very unusual circumstance, if you did not file a return for the correct year because your income was too low, you need to contact the Social Security Administration. Someone there can tell you how to proceed with convincing Social Security that you did not, in fact, file.

Another twist on this could be that Social Security used the correct year, but not the correct return. In other words, perhaps you amended your return since you originally filed, and your amended return would lower or eliminate the premium surcharge. If this is the case, you need to contact Social Security and someone there will tell you how to prove to Social Security that you amended your return.

Another situation is that a life-changing event may have occurred to you or your spouse since the return was filed. Maybe Social Security did use the correct year to determine your premium surcharge, but since then your marital status has changed and/or your income was reduced such that the surcharge does not apply to you (or should be less than you were told it was). If your marital status has changed through marriage, death, divorce, or annulment, you may be able to eliminate or reduce your premium surcharge. For example, if your income remained the same and you got married to someone without much income, there may be no need for the surcharge any longer.

Even if your legal marital status did not change but you did not live with your spouse at any time during the year in question, this can affect the amount of your premium surcharge as you now don't have to use the disadvantageous "married, filing separately" category.

One other situation you should be aware of is a change due to specific events. For example, since you filed your tax return, your income may have become lower due to certain very specific events. The following specific events allow Social Security to recalculate your premium surcharge because of a decrease in income:

- You or your spouse stopped working. Perhaps you retired, were laid off, sold your business, or left a corporate board.

- Your (or your spouse's) work hours were reduced. Perhaps you are on partial trial retirement, or there is a work slowdown at your company.

- You or your spouse received less income from an income-producing property due to disaster or an event beyond your control. These situations could include a hurricane, tornado, flood, or destruction of livestock due to disease, fire, or theft.

- Your (or your spouse's) benefits from an insured pension plan stopped or were reduced. In this case, the plan must be insured by the Pension Benefit Guaranty Corporation (PBGC). Your pension may have stopped or was reduced because of the pension plan's failure, or perhaps you had elected an annuity of a fixed number of years rather than for a lifetime, and it has run its course.

What you should do is figure out from Table 6 or Table 7 (depending on your filing status) and the information that is in your Modified Adjusted Gross Income (MAGI) letter, if the change that occurred will affect your premium. For example, your joint income may have slipped from $174,000 to $168,000 because you now work fewer hours. This small change just happens to put you below the threshold for the extra premium for 2009.

If you get a predetermination letter and if any of these marital or income-lowering events have occurred, it might lower your premium. Follow the instructions in the letter and let the Social Security Administration know about the changes. However, instead of calling as the letter suggests, contact the Social Security Administration in writing as these determinations are still fairly new to the Social Security employees.

Your predetermination letter will seem to say that you have only ten days from its date to do anything, but this is not necessarily true. Don't delay; let Social Security know as soon as you can, even if you were on vacation when the letter came in. Based on what information you give Social Security, it will give you an initial, formal decision that either changes your adjustment or does not.

When you get your initial determination letter or your cost-of-living increase letter, you should know that these are both final decisions and will go into effect unless you appeal them. You have only 60 days to appeal in writing. Note that you can ask for a new determination when you get your cost-of-increase letter rather than appealing, but my advice is to appeal. For more information on appeals, see Chapter 14.

One question that people always ask is how a significant one-time boost to your income re-

lates to your premium surcharge. For example, say in a given tax year that you sold off stock in which you had big gains, you cashed your Individual Retirement Account (IRA), or you converted an IRA into a Roth IRA. The bad news is that these one-time boosts to your income do count as income and do cause this extra income to be included in the MAGI calculation. Thus, a premium surcharge may go into effect for you, or your premium surcharge amount may increase, two years from the tax year during which you reported the boost. The good news is that your MAGI will be recalculated for the next year, and if you don't have any upward jags to your income, the premium surcharge may be eliminated or reduced.

Another situation is retroactivity. The general rule is that when Social Security adds a premium surcharge, it will apply it to the whole year in question. For example, suppose Social Security used the wrong tax year to determine your 2010 premium surcharge — say 2007 instead of 2008. You bring Social Security your tax return for 2008 sometime during 2010 and it shows you should have no premium surcharge for 2010. Even if Social Security has changed your premium amount, and you have had to pay it, once it decides that the premium surcharge should not have applied, you will receive the difference between the correct amount and what you already paid for that year.

Again, do not delay; when you get a MAGI letter, promptly address the matter. Not only are there time limits in which you may make your appeal (the standard 60 days), but the Social Security Administration will not make a correction retroactive into a prior year; in other words, it will look only at the year in question.

There is one exception to this rule. When you receive a notice during the last three months of the affected premium year, you may request a correction for the affected premium year until

March 31 of the following year. You may also make that request later, but only if there is good cause to extend the date.

9.3 Paying your premium amounts

Most people will have to pay the Part B premium on their own (and the Part A one, if they have premium Part A; see Chapter 2 for more on Part A). If you are getting a Social Security, Railroad Retirement payment, or federal retirement pension, the premium will be taken out of your monthly payment automatically. If you are not receiving these payments, you will be billed for your premium by the Medicare Premium Collection Center.

Your notice will typically ask you to pay for three months at a time. What it does not tell you is that you may ask to be billed monthly instead of quarterly. You can call Medicare to arrange monthly billing.

Be advised that if for some reason you miss paying your Part B premiums, you will have a chance to rectify the situation and keep your coverage. Your premium notice will tell you that your Part B will terminate if you do not pay by the due date. You will always be mailed a delinquency second notice and, as your grace period ends, a third notice. The timing of these notices and the grace period differs according to whether you are billed quarterly or monthly. You need to pay attention to these notices and get your premiums paid, because if you are terminated, your opportunity to re-enroll is limited to the general enrollment period, and your premiums may be penalized.

10. Information about Your Medicare Number and Card

Sometimes the Social Security Administration will change your Medicare number. This will happen if you have been entitled to Social Security and Medicare on someone else's account and then you become entitled on your own account. For example, you may have been entitled as a widow and received Medicare at age 60. Perhaps you worked after this point and earned enough quarters to become entitled on your own account. If so, you will be entitled on your own account, and your Medicare number will change. Be sure that any health care providers who have been using your old number begin to use your new one.

Your Medicare number (sometimes called your Health Insurance Claim Number) is a nine-digit number followed by one or two letters. Note that if the letter is "A" it does not mean you have Part A, or if it's "B" it doesn't mean you have Part B. What parts you are entitled to are shown underneath the phrase "Is Entitled To" on your Medicare card.

Note that while your red, white, and blue Medicare card will show whether or not you are entitled to Part A and/or Part B and the effective dates of each, sometimes these dates are different. It will not show whether you have Part C or D.

If you are enrolled in a Part D, a stand-alone drug plan, you will get a separate card. (All Original Medicare beneficiaries who enroll in Part D will be in a stand-alone drug plan, as will some Medicare Advantage managed care or health plan beneficiaries.) Always show this when you are getting your prescriptions filled or renewed at the pharmacy.

If you are enrolled in a Medicare Advantage managed care or health plan (i.e., Part C), you will get a separate card from your health care or managed care plan. It's very important that you show this card and not your red, white, and blue card when you get care. This is because your provider will assume you are in Original Medicare if you don't show your plan's card, and this will cause billing problems for your provider and you. You probably won't have a separate card for your Part D if you sign up for Part C — your Part C card will usually cover the things a Part D card would.

If you lose your Medicare card, you can get it replaced by calling Medicare, by calling the Social Security Administration, or by going to their websites. Note that it will probably take almost a month for you to get your new card, so if you need proof that you have Medicare in a hurry, you should visit your local Social Security office. If you get benefits from the Railroad Retirement Board, you will need to call the Board if you lose your card.

Never let anyone else use your Medicare card, and keep the number as safe as you would a credit card number. Identity theft experts say not to carry your card routinely, as identity thieves may get your Social Security number through your Medicare number.

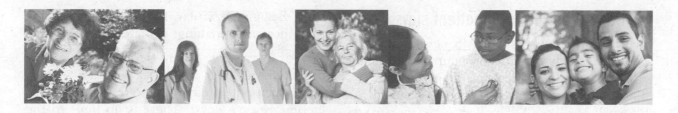

2
Part A

Part A is by far the most straightforward part of Medicare to understand. The vast majority of beneficiaries get Part A automatically and never have to think of whether they should keep it; they have already paid for it through years of deductions made from their (and their employer's) payroll or, if they were self-employed, from taxes paid every year.

Part A covers only four services and they all deal with acute care:

• Hospital inpatient stays

• Some Skilled Nursing Facility (SNF) stays

• Home health care

• Hospice care

Part A is designed as a progressive benefit. For example, the typical expectation is that you will experience an acute medical crisis requiring hospitalization, possibly including surgery or some other significant medical intervention; followed by a lesser level of inpatient care in a Skilled Nursing Facility; followed further by additional therapy and recovery care in the home setting. Part A does not pay for SNF care unless you have been hospitalized, and the same is true

for the home health benefit. (However, if you have Part B, you can get home health care without a hospital stay.) Hospice care is a stand-alone Part A benefit — you can get it with or without having used any of the other benefits.

Note that Part A pays only for a facility's charges and does not pay for doctor's visits and surgeon's fees (you need Part B to cover those costs).

1. Hospital Inpatient Stays

For most people, hospital inpatient stays won't be very complicated provided you have Part A of Medicare — at least not financially. This is because your only liability will probably be your inpatient deductible, which in 2010 is $1,100, and you will be discharged within 60 days before any additional liability accrues to you. Medicare data shows us that close to 99 percent of stays are 60 days or less, so you likely need not concern yourself with further details. In fact, the average stay is six days! Except for a few exceptions, which will be discussed in this chapter, Medicare will often take care of the hospital's bill — so Part A is excellent insurance.

1.1 Benefit period for inpatient stays

Medicare structures its Part A benefits uniquely. Medicare mostly depends on your being admitted to an inpatient hospital. This structure is called the *benefit period* (sometimes known as the "spell of illness"). The Part A benefit period begins when you are first admitted to a hospital as an inpatient, and it generally continues until you have not been confined to a hospital or an SNF for at least 60 calendar days. This is true even if Medicare isn't paying for your stay.

Suppose you are admitted to a hospital and stay 8 days before being transferred into a Skilled Nursing Facility for a week. Your next benefit period will begin 60 days after you are discharged from the Skilled Nursing Facility. However, if you are again admitted to a hospital or a Skilled Nursing Facility within those 60 days — for any reason, even if it is not related to the reason you went in before — your benefit period is continued. You don't have to pay the deductible again if you are hospitalized within 60 days, but the number of days of care Medicare will pay for is limited by what you already used.

Once you pay your Part A inpatient deductible (in 2010 it is $1,100), Medicare's response will be as follows:

- Your first 60 days of care paid for in full by Medicare.

- For the next 30 days (i.e., days 61 to 90 of your stay), you have to pay one-quarter of the deductible (i.e., $275) for each day.

- For the next 60 days (i.e., days 91 to 150) you have to pay one-half of the deductible, or $550, for each day.*

- Beginning on day 151, Medicare no longer pays anything; you are on your own.

For every new benefit period, you pay the deductible all over again, but you get a completely new set of days of care (except for your lifetime reserve days). There is no limit to the number of benefit periods to which you are entitled.

The benefit period works the same no matter what type of hospital you are in (e.g., community hospital, tertiary hospital, rehabilitation hospital), as long as you're an inpatient. However, there is an exception: If you are in a stand-alone psychiatric hospital, you get a maximum of 190 days of care in a lifetime. The usual benefit period rules for deductibles and coinsurance days apply here too: after you have 190 days of care in this type of hospital at any point as a Medicare beneficiary, Medicare stops paying. This applies only to psychiatric hospitals, and not to days you spend in the psychiatric unit of a community hospital.

As with all care given by an institution, Medicare has to certify that a hospital meets Medicare standards. By law, if certain accrediting organizations (e.g., Joint Commission) approve a hospital, Medicare will certify it.

Note that if you are in a Medicare Advantage managed care or health plan, you may not be able to choose any hospital you want. You may be restricted to ones in your plan's network, or your plan may even own its very own hospital.

1.2 Medicare hospital benefits

Medicare will pay for just about every aspect of your hospital stay, except for the following:

---

*Note: For days 91 to 150, each Medicare Part A beneficiary gets a once-in-a lifetime reserve of days — 60 days in all — which Medicare will add to the end of your stay when you run out of hospital days. Remember, this is once-in-a lifetime, so if you have used your reserved days during another stay, Medicare won't cover you for the additional stay again. You pay half the deductible for each of these days ($550 per day in 2010).

- Private duty nursing

- Separate charges for phone, TV, Internet connection — but note that most hospitals include these charges in the room rate, which *is* covered

- Private rooms (unless staying in a private room is medically necessary, or the hospital only has private rooms)

- The first three pints of blood you use. Medicare has a separate deductible for blood. It will not pay for the first three pints of blood you use in a calendar year. This is Medicare's attempt to help ensure the blood supply is replenished. However, if you can pre-donate, or get friends or family to donate in your name, hospitals can't charge you for this. The hospital can't charge you if it gets the blood from a blood bank at no charge. However, if the hospital has to pay for the blood, and you have not already met your blood deductible for the year, the hospital can bill you.

All other hospital charges are covered, including your Computerized Axial Tomography (CAT) scans and diagnostic tests (even if you were transported to another facility for them), lab charges (even if your specimen was sent to an independent lab), nurses, therapists, the operating and recovery room, intensive care, medicines and IVs, and any device that gets implanted in you (e.g., a pacemaker or artificial hip). Even treatments you may typically be paying for under Part B are covered. For example, if you normally get several dialysis treatments every week in a stand-alone dialysis facility under Part B, and you have a heart attack and are admitted to hospital, your dialysis will be paid for under Part A while you are an inpatient.

Sometimes, if you have a planned admission (e.g., scheduled surgery), the hospital will ask you to come to its lab, X-ray department, or diagnostic clinic for preadmission testing. Other times, you may get diagnostic tests as an outpatient and later be admitted as an inpatient. If either of these situations happens within three days of your admission, the hospital has to include the charges for these tests on your inpatient bill, even though you had them as an outpatient. This is good for you because they will not increase your hospital bill. If it is for a planned admission, try to get your tests at the hospital you will be admitted to, and within the three-day time frame. This three-day rule also applies to non-diagnostic procedures you get from the hospital if they are directly related to your subsequent admission.

1.3 Special notes on Medicare hospital coverage

There are always some questions that surround your admission and discharge which are gray areas, and it's helpful for you to know a little about these issues.

If you are admitted or discharged from the hospital in an ambulance, and this trip is otherwise covered, this will not be included in your bill for your inpatient stay. Ambulance service is separate from hospital stays and is covered under Part B. As a result, it will be separately billed, with responsibility lying on you to pay for the Part B coinsurance.

The hospital will sometimes give you a modest, transitional supply of medication or IV upon discharge so there isn't an interruption to your treatment. You are responsible for the cost of these items once you are discharged.

Also important to note here is the issue of hospital admission. Suppose you go to a hospital and the hospital just doesn't know whether you should be admitted or not. The hospital may put you in an observation room or hold you in the emergency room. No strict limits apply to this;

Medicare says these periods should be limited to 24 hours and with rare exceptions should not exceed 48 hours.

2. Skilled Nursing Facility (SNF) Care

Skilled Nursing Facility is often abbreviated as SNF. It is a term that is primarily associated with the Medicare program. SNF is a fairly intense level of care and rehabilitation and is usually provided in a place that mostly gives "regular" nursing home care. Sometimes Medicare will refer to Skilled Nursing Facility care as "extended care," not because it goes on for an extended period of time, but because it's an extension of hospital care.

2.1 Qualifying for a stay

For Medicare to pay for your stay in a Skilled Nursing Facility (SNF), you have to meet seven requirements. The first three requirements are technical:

- You must be discharged from a Medicare-covered hospital inpatient stay that lasted at least three nights in a row.

- Your SNF admission must be based on a condition that you had treated in the hospital.

- You have to be admitted into the SNF within 30 calendar days of your discharge from the hospital.*

You can see this Medicare Part A benefit is closely tied to inpatient hospital care. You should understand that if you were *not* in the hospital for the requisite three consecutive nights, or you were out of the hospital for more than 30 days before you were admitted to an SNF, Medicare will not pay for your SNF care.

You should be aware that if you were kept overnight in a hospital for observation (and not actually admitted), this does *not* count toward the three-night hospital inpatient stay requirement.

As an aside, some Medicare Advantage managed care or health (Part C) plans waive the three-night requirement, and your plan may pay for your care in an SNF after a shorter hospital stay.

In addition to the three technical requirements, you have to meet four other medical requirements. These are strict requirements because Medicare wants to avoid paying for custodial care. The four medical requirements include when:

- Your physician determines that you need this level of care.

- You need skilled nursing care or skilled therapy services (or a combination thereof) on a daily basis. (Note: Medicare does not require you to get therapy services on the weekend.)

- The services can only be given to you as an inpatient in an SNF.

- The services you receive must be reasonable and necessary to treat your medical condition, and reasonable in terms of duration and quantity.

You need to go to a Medicare-certified SNF. Most nursing homes qualify as a certified facility, and your hospital discharge planners or social workers will help you find a qualified facility. Some hospitals have an SNF on their campus

---

*Note: An exception allows your admission to take place after 30 days if, at the time of your hospital discharge, it would be medically inappropriate to begin an active course of treatment in an SNF and a predictable time exists as to when a covered stay will be needed. The example Medicare gives is a patient with a hip fracture discharged from the hospital. As therapy cannot normally be given for a month or so until healing takes place and the hip can bear weight, a predictable time exists for admission to a SNF for covered services, which in this example could be physical therapy. If, in this example, admission took place 35 days after the hospital discharge, that would be an acceptable exception to the 30-day rule.

or in the same building as the hospital. In many rural areas, hospitals are allowed to switch you from hospital care to an SNF care while you are in the same bed!

You can see the requirements for admission are fairly high. If you are admitted, you will be formally assessed, probably by your fifth day in the facility, or it may be as late as your eighth day.

2.2 What Medicare covers in a Skilled Nursing Facility

Skilled Nursing Facilities (SNFs) are required to have available a wide array of services to rehabilitate you and improve your condition. These services include:

- **Skilled nursing care:** This includes the development and evaluation of your care plan, intravenous feedings, intramuscular injections, suprapubic catheter insertions, intravenous feedings, nasopharyngeal and tracheotomy aspiration, and many other skilled services.

- **Physical therapy:** This may include an assessment of your physical condition including your range of motion, strength, or coordination; therapeutic exercise planning; gait training; establishment of an exercise maintenance program; specialized baths (e.g., whirlpools) where complications such as an open wound are involved; and heat treatments.

- **Occupational therapy:** This includes assisting you in relearning daily routines such as dressing, eating, grooming, housekeeping, and helping with balance and coordination.

- **Speech-language pathology:** This includes having you relearn speech (e.g., stroke victims). It can include the services of audiologists.

- **Dietary counseling:** This helps to ensure you get the best nutrition in light of your condition.

- **Medical social services:** These services help you adjust to the social and emotional issues of your illness and condition. These services can also help with locating possible financial assistance as well as finding community resources for you at discharge.

An SNF offers a high level of care. Nursing care in an SNF must be given by Registered Nurses (RNs) or Licensed Practical Nurses (LPNs), and the therapies given by the appropriate certified therapists. Social services are provided by Medical Social Workers (MSWs). Some of your personal care (e.g., bathing) will be provided by certified nurse assistants.

An important aspect of the therapy you get in the facility will be that it must have the expectation that your condition will improve materially and in a reasonable and somewhat predictable period of time. Again, this requirement is one Medicare uses to avoid paying for custodial care. If your condition does not improve in spite of the therapy, your care will be deemed custodial and Medicare will stop covering your stay.

Note that a lot of the skilled care mentioned here involves training you in how to administer your own care; for example, colostomy care or performing repetitive, therapeutic exercises. The training may be the most important care you receive as it will enable you to deal with your condition after you have been discharged.

When you are in an SNF, Medicare will pay for the following:

- The full costs of your first 20 days in the facility.

- For the next 80 days, Medicare will pay for everything but $137.50 a day (in 2010), which is one-eighth of the hospital deductible.

- Medicare does not pay for anything after the 100th day.

It may help knowing that the average Medicare length of stay in an SNF is about 35 days, so chances are you will have a number of coinsurance days at which you are responsible for the $137.50 per day after the first 20 days.

Medicare will pay for just about everything for your SNF stay, including your medicine and any kind of medical equipment you need, with the same exceptions as with hospitals (e.g., SNFs will not pay for luxuries such as separate TV or phone charges and private nursing). Note that Medicare Part A will not cover visits by your physician to the SNF.

Although SNF stays are paid under a comprehensive prospective payment system, and even though the purpose of this system is to bundle all the costs together, some of the treatments you get while in an SNF will not be covered in your facility bill. These are fairly intensive services and generally involve taking you outside the facility for specialized procedures in a hospital or other clinical settings. Such services include kidney dialysis, cardiac catheterization, Magnetic Resonance Imaging (MRI), CAT scan, angiography, and radiation therapy, as well as use of a hospital emergency room or an operating room when these are needed. Medicare Part B will cover these, but you will be responsible for the coinsurance.

If you need ambulance services, many of these will not be bundled in your bill and you will have to pay for them separately. These services include transporting you to be admitted to or discharged from the SNF, and if the ambulance service is needed, transporting you to a hospital (e.g., for outpatient surgery) or to a dialysis treatment. Part B will cover these.

It may be necessary to discharge you from the SNF for a brief time (e.g., should you need to be hospitalized overnight). In this case, Medicare will not pay for your SNF to hold your bed so you can be certain to be readmitted to it and not somewhere else. You may make private arrangements with the facility for a hold, if you are willing to pay for it.

2.3 Benefit period for a Skilled Nursing Facility

This section will help you understand how your Part A benefits work in the time frame soon after you are either discharged from a Skilled Nursing Facility (SNF), or when your level of care in the facility no longer qualifies as skilled.

Medicare will cover your care and your benefit period will continue if, within 30 calendar days, you are readmitted to an SNF. Similarly, you will be covered if your care in a facility that you did not leave changes so it becomes skilled. How much of it Medicare will pay for depends on how many SNF days of care you have left in your benefit period.

Medicare will not pay for your SNF care if you are readmitted to an SNF 30 to 60 calendar days after your initial admission, because there was a lapse in this type of care for more than 30 days during this benefit period.

If a full 60 calendar days pass and you have not received SNF or hospital care, your benefit period expires. You become eligible for a new benefit period when you are first admitted to a hospital, or in unusual circumstances, to an SNF. If you have an inpatient stay of three or more days, you will again be eligible for SNF care.

The following are some examples of how the Part A benefit period works:

Example 1

Suppose you are hospitalized for a week then discharged directly into a Skilled Nursing Facility (SNF) for a two-week stay (i.e., 14 days).

In this case, your benefit period begins when you are admitted to the hospital. Medicare will pay all but your inpatient deductible. As your stay there was longer than three nights, and you went right into skilled nursing care, it will also pay for all of your SNF care. You will be responsible for a total of $1,100 (the 2010 inpatient deductible).

At this point in your benefit period you have —

- satisfied the hospital inpatient deductible,
- 53 days of full hospital care left,
- 30 days of $275 coinsurance days left,
- 60 days of $550 coinsurance lifetime reserve days left,
- 6 days of full SNF care left, and
- 80 $137.50 coinsurance days of SNF care left.

Example 2

Suppose you are hospitalized for ten days for a stroke then you are discharged to your home as no SNF beds are available. Three weeks later you are admitted to an SNF for physical and speech rehabilitation from your stroke. You are there for 40 days.

Your benefit period begins with your hospitalization, and Medicare will pay all but your hospital inpatient deductible. As you entered an SNF within 30 days of your discharge from the hospital, and for the same condition, Medicare will pay for your first 20 days of care there in full. It will pay for all but $137.50 a day (SNF coinsurance) for the remaining 20 days. You will be responsible for $137.50 a day for a total of $2,750 ($137.50 x 20) for coinsurance, and $1,100 for the hospital deductible, for a total of $3,850.

At this point in your benefit period you have —

- satisfied the hospital inpatient deductible,
- 50 days of full hospital care left,
- 30 days of $275 coinsurance days left,
- 60 days of $550 coinsurance lifetime reserve days left,
- 0 days of full SNF care left, and
- 60 days of $137.50 coinsurance SNF care left.

Example 3

Following a stroke, suppose you are admitted to a community hospital for a 12-day stay and then are transferred to a rehabilitation hospital for a 50-day stay. You are discharged to your home, but four weeks later are admitted to an SNF for additional rehabilitation. You are discharged from there to your home after 17 days. Twenty-five days later you return to another SNF for intensive inhalation therapy following a severe bout of pneumonia. You are discharged after five weeks (i.e., 35 days).

Your benefit period begins with your hospitalization. You will pay the inpatient deductible, and Medicare will pay for all the rest except the last two days in the rehab hospital. This is because you used all your 60 full inpatient days. You will have to pay $550, that is, two days of the $275 per day (61 to 90 days coinsurance). The fact that you were transferred from one hospital to another is not relevant. Your liability for your hospital stays is the $1,100 deductible plus the $550, which equals $1,650.

As far as your SNF care, your first admission was within 30 days of your hospital discharge and for the same condition so it will be covered. Medicare will pay for everything. Your second admission is covered by Medicare because it occurred within 30 days of your previous SNF discharge. This is true even though it was for a different condition. It must be the *same* condition as your hospitalization for your *first* SNF stay, but *not* for a readmission to a SNF. It is irrelevant if it is the same or a different SNF. Medicare will cover all your days in the first SNF, but you will be liable to the second SNF for 32 days of $137.50 coinsurance days of the 35 days you spent there; this amounts to $4,400. If you add this to your hospital liability of $1,650, your total liability is $6,050.

At this point in your benefit period you have —

- satisfied the hospital inpatient deductible,
- 0 days of full hospital care left,
- 28 days of $275 coinsurance days left,
- 60 days of $550 coinsurance lifetime reserve days left,
- 0 days of full SNF care left, and
- 48 days of $137.50 coinsurance SNF care left.

By going through these examples you get the idea that the benefit period rules both dictate what stays will be covered and determine the coinsurance dollars, if any, for which you are responsible.

You should note that if, in Example 3, your second SNF admission occurred more than 30 days after your first stay's discharge, Medicare will not pay for the care in the facility because too much time elapsed after your first discharge, but your benefit period will continue. This situation will also occur if you exhaust all your hospital days but are still in the hospital. However, this is an extremely rare situation.

You may want to go through these same three examples assuming that all this occurs without a renewal of the benefit period; in other words, assume you are readmitted to the hospital within 60 days of your discharge from your last SNF stay.

For example 1, the situation does not change.

For example 2, you do not pay the inpatient deductible again. (You pay it once in a benefit period no matter how many admissions you have.) Medicare pays the rest of the hospital bill and you have 43 days of full hospital care left.

The second Skilled Nursing Facility (SNF) stay is covered as it meets all the requirements. (Again, a benefit period does *not* limit the number of hospital or SNF admissions, it limits the number of days Medicare will pay in full, in part, or not at all.) However, with this second stay you will have the first 6 days covered in full and the last 34 days paid for except for the $137.50 per day coinsurance. You will be liable for a total of $4,675 (i.e., 34 days at $137.50 per day).

At this point in your benefit period you have —

- satisfied the inpatient deductible,
- 43 days of full hospital care left,
- 30 days of $275 coinsurance days left,
- 60 days of $550 coinsurance lifetime reserve days left,
- 0 days of full SNF care left, and
- 46 days of $137.50 coinsurance SNF care left.

In example 3, you do not pay the inpatient deductible again. Medicare pays the bill from the community hospital (i.e., 12 days), and it pays all of the first 31 days of the rehab hospital stay (at which point you have used all 43 remaining full hospital days). Medicare will pay all of the remaining 19 days at the rehab hospital except for the $275 per day coinsurance. You will owe the rehab hospital $5,225 (i.e., 19 x $275).

Both SNF stays are covered as each meet all the requirements. The first stay will be paid for except for the $137.50 per day coinsurance for each of the 17 days. You will be liable for a total of $2,337.50 ($137.50 x 17). The second stay will be paid for except for the $137.50 per day coinsurance for each of the remaining 29 days of coinsurance days left to you (remember that you get only 80 of these per benefit period), or for a total of $3,987.50 (i.e., $137.50 x 29), and you will have to pay for the remaining 6 days by yourself.

At this point in your benefit period you have —

- satisfied the inpatient deductible,
- 0 days of full hospital care left,
- 11 days of $275 coinsurance days left,
- 60 days of $550 coinsurance lifetime reserve days left,
- 0 days of full SNF care left, and
- 0 days of $137.50 coinsurance SNF care left.

Note that in this last scenario that your stay was so long that you ran out of SNF coinsurance days and are still there for six days in which you are liable for the full payment. Three very important points must be made about this:

- Just because you run out of coinsurance days and Medicare stops paying for your care, this does not mean that you are no longer a Medicare beneficiary in that institution, whether it's a hospital or an SNF. As long as you are receiving a covered level of care, Medicare reimbursement

rules still apply, and your liability is determined by what Medicare would have paid for the stay using its rules — not whatever the hospital or SNF wants to charge you, which is usually much more.

- You are also sheltered by all the Medicare rules governing your rights and protections as an inpatient, as well as your quality of care, so you can invoke your rights whenever you want.

If you have Part B of Medicare, it will pay for your diagnostic tests and treatments that are covered by Part B, even though you are an inpatient that Medicare is no longer paying for. These Part B services are called *ancillary services*.

If you do get admitted to a covered Medicare stay at an SNF, your spell of illness will expire —

- when you are discharged and you are not readmitted to a covered stay in either an SNF or a hospital for 60 days in a row; or
- if you remain in a SNF, but you do not get skilled care there for 60 days in a row.

Note the quite unusual but possible situation that if you remain in an SNF and you are receiving skilled care, your benefit period will continue even though Medicare is not paying for it (because you ran out of your 100 SNF days). If you remain in the facility, you will be in a limbo situation until your skilled care ends for 60 days in a row.

3. Home Health Care

Home health care is the next progression of care in the Part A benefits. Home health care is good for the Medicare program itself, because it's a way for the program to keep you away from very expensive inpatient care. In many respects, your recovery can be aided if you are in a familiar home setting as opposed to an institutional one.

The home health care benefit has some unique aspects to it. For example, you pay nothing for home health care visits, which means no deductible, coinsurance, or co-payment. Part A or Part B will pay for it. If you have Part A and are in a benefit period (normally this comes after a three-night hospital stay), Part A will generally pay for these visits (up to 100 in that period). If you don't have Part A, and you have Part B, Part B will pay for it. There are no set limits as to how many visits Medicare will pay for under Part B, and if your Part A visits run out, Part B will take over. It makes no difference to you if Part A or Part B pays, so, in a way, this is one of the easiest Medicare benefits to learn.

3.1 Home health-care benefits

You do not have to have a qualifying stay in a hospital or Skilled Nursing Facility to receive home health-care benefits, but you do have to meet the following requirements:

- You have to be homebound.
- You must require part-time skilled nursing care, physical therapy, speech-language pathology, or continue to need occupational therapy.
- You have to be under the care of a doctor, and the doctor has to certify that you need care in the home and approve your plan of care.

3.1a Homebound care

Homebound care may apply to you if it is a considerable and taxing effort for you to leave your home, and that normally you cannot leave your home unassisted (i.e., you need help from another person or with equipment to aid you). Medicare does understand that even though it is difficult, there are a number of instances in which you actually leave your home but are still considered homebound. These

include trips on an infrequent basis or of a short duration, for example to:

- Go to any provider of medical services (e.g., doctor's office).
- Attend a religious service or a funeral.
- Obtain personal care (e.g., haircut).
- Participate in adult day care. This does not mean merely going to the local senior center, but some actual treatment (i.e., rehabilitative, psychosocial, or medical) in a licensed adult day care program.
- Attend an important family occasion (e.g., holiday dinner).
- Do something less formal (e.g., neighbor takes you for a drive).

Your inability to leave home unassisted might be due to a physical cause or mental condition. However, Medicare is always cautious not to pay for or cover custodial care. If your trips appear to show that you could reasonably receive your care outside the home, you would not be considered homebound. For example, if an aged person leaves home infrequently because of feebleness or insecurity caused by advancing age, the person would not be considered homebound simply because of his or her reluctance to go out, or because it takes an extra effort to do so.

However, if you have had an onset of illness or a real deterioration in your condition, and it is now very difficult for you to get out, you will probably qualify as homebound, at least for a while. You have to be in your home to get home health services. For instance, if you are discharged from a Medicare-covered Skilled Nursing Facility stay, but elect to remain in the facility, you can't get home health services there because it is not your home or residence. Along similar lines, if you live in a group home or some sort of institution that is required to provide your care, you may be in your home, but

Medicare home health will not cover you as another party is responsible for your care.

3.1b Skilled nursing or therapy care

In order to receive home health-care benefits, you must require part-time skilled nursing care, physical therapy, speech-language pathology, or occupational therapy. This is actually a very definite requirement that not only specifies the explicit services you must be getting, but it also places limitations on them from several angles. What it means is that to get home health care from Medicare, you must be getting the following:

- **Skilled nursing services:** Nursing services are covered only if required on a part-time or intermittent basis. Medicare defines part-time or intermittent care as skilled nursing or home health-aide services which, combined, must total less than 8 hours per day and 28 hours per week, with some exceptions of up to 35 hours a week. And, in general, may not be more than six days a week. If you require more care than this, you will not be covered. Those who require a high level of services won't be covered under Medicare; Medicare feels that these beneficiaries should be getting their care in a Skilled Nursing Facility.

- **Physical therapy, speech-language pathology, or occupational therapy:** Physical therapy and speech-language pathology are both covered under home health-care benefits. However, if you require occupational therapy, it must initially be accompanied by *one of* skilled nursing services, speech-langauge pathology, or physical therapy in order to qualify. If you continue to require occupational therapy after your need for the other services ceases, your occupational therapy is still covered; however, if you only need occupational therapy without the accompaniment of any of the other services to begin with, you are not covered under Medicare.

3.1c Doctor certified home care

The third requirement of receiving homebound health-care benefits is that your doctor has to certify that you need care in the home, and he or she must approve your plan of care.

Medicare's general approach to its benefits is that physicians should be the decision makers in deciding what kind of care you should receive and in what amounts. That's why your physician signs your hospital admissions and discharges, and gets involved in your home health care. What typically happens is that your doctor tells a home health agency that you need care, and the agency will send a nurse to evaluate you. If the agency agrees that you qualify, it will create a plan of care based on its evaluation of your condition and what services you need, and ask your doctor to approve it.

The way the home health benefit works is that it's grouped in 60-calendar-day episodes of care. Your initial plan will span this entire period. The reason for this is that, like most Part A services (even though Part B may actually pay), payments by Medicare for your care to a home health agency are determined by a prospective payment system. More specifically, your condition is assessed in great detail by a nurse or therapist and recorded on something called an Outcome and Assessment Information Set. Based on all this information, your home health agency will be paid a set amount for your care.

3.2 Additional home health-care benefits

Besides the benefits listed in the previous section (i.e., skilled nursing, physical therapy, speech-language pathology, and occupational therapy), there are other types of services as well:

- **Home health aide services:** These are aides who provide assistance (not skilled nursing), such as bathing, feeding, dressing, and helping you to the toilet. These services have to be intermittent. The home health benefit will not pay for 24-hour nurse aides.

- **Medical social services:** These services include counseling to help you cope with the social and mental issues related to your condition, including identifying community resources and financial assistance.

- **All routine and nonroutine medical supplies that are needed:** Routine medical supplies may include alcohol swabs and incontinence briefs, while nonroutine may include sterile dressings, ostomy bags, syringes, and blood glucose or urine monitoring strips.

- **Durable medical equipment:** This can include hospital beds, wheelchairs, potties, and devices to help you in and out of bed. The equipment may be directly supplied by a home health agency or the agency may arrange for a supplier to send the equipment to your home and set it up. No matter how it's supplied, you have to pay 20 percent coinsurance on it, even if your home health care is being covered under Part A. (This is the only time you pay a 20 percent coinsurance in Part A.) The home health agency does not have to provide under the general home health benefit those supplies that are covered under the durable medical equipment benefit; these are covered, but as part of that benefit, and you have to pay coinsurance on them.

- **Osteoporosis drugs:** The home health benefit covers osteoporosis drugs for female beneficiaries who have broken a bone and are under a home health plan of care when these specific shots are injected by one of the agency's staff. The cost of the shot itself (i.e., the osteoporosis drug) is covered only under Part B, even when the cost of the visit to give you the shot is covered by Part A. The beneficiary is responsible for the Part B deductible and coinsurance for the shot, but the home health benefit will pay the full cost of the visit itself. Under some circumstances, the plan of care can be established for the sole purpose of administering this shot.

Medicare must provide these services, even when there is someone available to the patient to do them, such as a capable spouse or family member. The home health agency must perform the services unless that person is fully capable and clearly indicates that he or she will perform the needed services. You should be aware that if for some reason the home health agency can't give you one of these covered services in your home, it must take you to where you can get the appropriate service (e.g., hospital rehab clinic). In this situation, you are not responsible for the hospital fees; the home health agency must pay for this service, as well as for the cost of transportation to and from the hospital.

The home health benefit will not pay for the following:

- Prescription drugs (although the visit to inject you with an osteoporosis drug is covered, as noted above);

- Homemaker services, such as cleaning, shopping, and washing clothes (please note that a home health aide can perform these services if they are incidental, which means the aide visit is needed in and of itself to give you a health-related service covered in your plan of care); and

- Food, except under the durable medical equipment benefit, such as parenteral (intravenous feeding) and enteral (tube feeding) supplies.

This does not mean that you can't get these kinds of services from your agency, but the agency has to be crystal clear with you about what it will provide and how much you will have to pay for these services. This also has to be in writing from the agency.

Because you are in a somewhat vulnerable situation when in home health care (since your care is given in your home and not in an institution that is visited by outside inspectors), there is a special way that you can complain about your home health care if you feel that something is amiss, such as poor quality services, overly short visits, lack of responsiveness to your needs, and so forth. You can contact the State Home Health hotline, a toll-free number connected to your state health-care licensing agency. Your home health agency must give you this number when it begins care for you. Alternatively, you can call the Quality Improvement Organization that serves your state.

One final note on home health care: When your home health agency wants to discontinue your care, it has to give you notice at least two days before it ends the visits. This formal notice is called a Notice of Medicare Provider Noncoverage. This document will tell you when your covered services will end, how much you will have to pay the agency if you want the services to be continued, and how to get a fast-track appeal, as well as your right to get a more detailed notice about why your services are ending.

4. Hospice Care

The fourth type of care available under Part A is hospice care, which is chosen by a patient who has decided that it is preferable to face death in as much comfort and dignity as possible rather than to continue direct treatment for a terminal disease. These patients are often those with cancer, emphysema, Alzheimer's, AIDS, or those suffering from an advanced degenerative disease,

in some cases of a neuromuscular or cardiovascular nature.

There are only a few requirements for choosing to have hospice care. First, you have to have Part A of Medicare. Your physician as well as the hospice's medical director must certify that you are terminally ill and that you have less than six months (usually) to live. You have to sign a statement that you want hospice care rather than routine medical care for your terminal illness. What is most important to know is what the benefit does and doesn't cover, as this is what you really need to know about it to consider it as an option.

The most important thing to know about hospice coverage is that when you choose this option, Medicare will no longer pay to treat the condition or illness leading to your death. So any therapeutic or curative service or treatment you receive that is designed to treat your terminal illness will not be covered. Opting for hospice care is a serious decision that should not be taken lightly.

You should also understand that you have the option, at any time, of leaving hospice coverage and seeking regular treatment. If it turns out that your illness is not terminal (medical diagnosis is not always an exact science), or if it goes into remission, then you must leave this coverage option. From the Medicare insurance point of view, going into a hospice is not an irrevocable choice.

4.1 What hospice care covers

If you choose hospice care, a hospice provider that you select will form an interdisciplinary team, which will work with you and your family to keep you as comfortable as possible and to assist you, your family, and your caregivers with your terminal illness. More specifically, a hospice will cover a wide array of medical services that Medicare always pays for. These services will be designed to relieve pain, alleviate distressing or irritating symptoms, and to prevent such symptoms from occurring to the extent possible. In the hospice setting, the emotional well-being as well as the physical are taken into consideration, in the case of both the patient and his or her family or caregivers: Counseling and respite services are available to the family and caregivers of the hospice patient.

The medical services included in hospice care include those that ordinarily would be used to treat or cure an illness, but in the hospice patient's case are used only to make him or her more comfortable. An example, while quite unusual, would be the use of radiation therapy not to cure a tumor, but to reduce its size where it is impinging on an organ and thus causing much discomfort.

In summary, the services provided by a hospice include those given by the following:

- Physicians

- Nurses

- Medical social workers

- Therapists (including their help in allowing you to maintain skills for daily living)

- Home health aides

Medicare will also cover the costs of durable medical equipment and medical supplies.

The hospice benefit will also pay for services not typically covered by Medicare, including the following:

- Some homemaker services, such as changing the bed and any light cleaning or laundering necessary for the comfort and cleanliness of the patient.

- Prescription drugs for symptom control and pain relief.

- Grief and loss counseling for both you and your family, which, at your option, may be given by a member of the clergy.

- Respite care, to some extent. Respite care occurs when the family is given a chance to rest from the personal care they give the patient. Typically, this involves taking the patient to a hospital, nursing home, or hospice facility for a few days. Only if the patient is admitted for respite care, Medicare will pay the patient's room and board charges, except for a 5 percent coinsurance charge. A stay of no more than five days is permitted at one time. However, in any particular hospice period of care, there is no limit on the number of these stays.

- Bereavement counseling, which is the counseling the survivors receive after a death. It can be given to them for up to a year from the time of death; this is an exception to the principle that Medicare benefits cease with death.

Your hospice provider may also help coordinate trained volunteers who perform a variety of tasks including companionship, help with transportation, and homemaker chores. The volunteer aspect of the hospice program is somewhat unique. While certainly there are many volunteers in hospitals and nursing homes, hospice volunteers are often those whose family members have died from a long illness, and they have unique and helpful perspectives to offer others undergoing the same experience.

As can be seen by the wide array of unique services available under the hospice option, critical to understanding it is the patient's plan of care. These plans are highly individualized depending on the condition and prognosis of the patient, the locale of the care, the family and/or caregiver resources available to help, and on the wishes and desires of the patient. It goes without saying that you and your family and caregivers, as well as your personal physician have a big say in formulating these plans. As conditions change, the plan can be changed too.

Hospice care is centered on home care, which most beneficiaries prefer, but in some cases this is not an option as family members or others are not available to help the patient. In these cases, if a beneficiary is placed in a nursing home or a hospice facility, Medicare will not pay the routine room and board charges for the facility, but it will pay for hospice services. If the patient's terminal care requires an inpatient stay because of the need to control extreme pain, then the inpatient costs will be covered provided that this inpatient care takes place in a Medicare certified hospital, Skilled Nursing Facility, or hospice facility.

Medicare will continue to cover care not related to your terminal illness. For example, a flu shot would be covered, or emergency treatment for a burn would be covered by Original Medicare. If you are in a Medicare Advantage managed care or health plan, its rules will apply.

It is a tricky thing about the hospice benefit to determine what it does and does not pay for. Ultimately, it will not pay for therapeutic care for a terminal illness. To understand this, the following excerpt from the Medicare hospice regulations discusses this difficult area with some grace:

> *It is important that the patient and family be educated before the start of care that hospice entails certain limits in the way care will be provided … among them being restrictions on obtaining care outside those [limits] provided or arranged for by the hospice and the patient's potential liability for care received without the hospice's involvement. It is particularly important that the patient and caregiver be instructed on what to do in a crisis or emergency.*

Consider the following example: Suppose a Medicare hospice patient is dying from emphysema. One evening, a family member who does not normally help care for her is the only one present when the patient has a sudden breathing crisis. The family member panics and calls 911, and has that patient transported to the local hospital for emergency room treatment. This treatment may not be covered, because the patient is being treated for something directly linked to her condition.

When you elect for the hospice option, Medicare is not supposed to pay for therapeutic intervention in the terminal condition, and this should not be paid by the hospice (although the regulation indicates in this one unusual instance it perhaps should). It is very important for the hospice to make sure that the caregivers understand what to do in case of a crisis or emergency. One requirement that a hospice has to satisfy is that it has to have a doctor or nurse available by phone 24 hours a day, seven days a week, to help deal with these problems.

Because of the special relationship between you and your personal physician, one exception to the general principle that only the hospice can give care related to your final illness is that you can continue to have your physician involved and working with the hospice on your plan of care, and specific physician level services, such as changing your pain medication. However, no curative services related to your terminal illness may be paid.

As far as payments, hospice care does require the beneficiary to pay in two instances:

- A co-payment of $5 for each prescription drug or pain medicine.

- A coinsurance payment of 5 percent for any inpatient respite care. However, a complicated formula usually limits your total coinsurance payments to no more than $1,100 in 2010, which as you may recognize is the Part A hospital inpatient deductible for that calendar year.

4.2 Other hospice issues

Another issue you must face if you take the hospice option is that if you truly decide not to seek any curative medical care, you may wish to cancel your insurance (e.g., Medigap). Remember, if you do, you won't have its protection if you get care for something not related to your terminal illness, and in case your disease goes into remission, you may not be able to get your insurance back. Again, this is a difficult decision as it may not be reversible.

If you do decide to take the hospice option, you will hear a lot about hospice "periods of care" of 90 days and 60 days and so forth. While your hospice provider needs to observe these carefully to allow the medical director to periodically recertify your need for hospice care, the benefit has been made so flexible that you can stay in hospice care indefinitely — there is no limitation as long as you are terminally ill and you continue to want this approach. Even if you decide to leave, or if your condition becomes nonterminal, you can always go back to hospice care at a later time; again, there is no limitation.

You don't really need to be concerned with all the varying periods of care, with one exception. In any given period of care, you can change hospice providers, but only once. If you do not feel that you are being well-served by your current hospice provider, and there is another, Medicare-certified hospice provider available, you can change once in that 90- or 60-day period. At any given time, only one hospice can be giving you care.

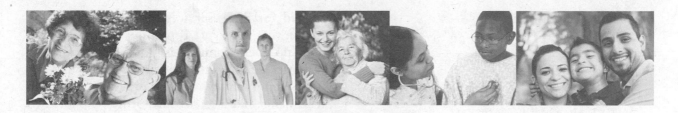

3
Part B: The Basics

Part B pays for an enormous variety of diagnostic, therapeutic, and preventative medical services. Because Part B covers so much, it is divided into three chapters for easier understanding. This chapter gives you some of the basics of Part B. Chapter 4 includes a detailed discussion of the benefits and services Part B covers. In Chapter 5, you will find information on the durable medical equipment that is covered under Part B.

1. Part B Providers

It helps to clarify this benefit by understanding that although many Part B services are given by individual practitioners such as your physician, much of it is also delivered by institutions such as hospital outpatient departments and emergency rooms, rehabilitation clinics, and ambulatory surgical centers. Indeed, this trend is growing through the universal shift in medical practice to give more services on an outpatient basis. The following list includes all the institutional providers that Medicare certifies to give Part B services:

- Hospitals
- Rural health clinics

- Skilled Nursing Facilities (SNFs)
- Federally qualified health centers
- Home health agencies
- Ambulatory surgical centers
- End-stage renal disease dialysis clinics
- Clinical laboratories
- Comprehensive outpatient rehab facilities
- Portable x-ray suppliers
- Community mental health centers

Health-care practitioners themselves are not certified by Medicare. Practitioners who may provide Part B services include:

- Physicians
- Certified registered nurse anesthetists
- Clinical social workers
- Anesthesiologist's assistants
- Physician assistants
- Certified nurse midwives
- Clinical nurse specialists

- Nurse practitioners
- Dentists
- Chiropractors
- Optometrists
- Podiatrists and surgical chiropodists
- Pharmacies
- Ambulance companies
- Orthotists and prosthetists
- Durable medical equipment suppliers
- Physical therapists
- Nutritionists
- Speech-language pathologists
- Occupational therapists
- Opticians
- Qualified audiologists

Through this listing you can see how wide the scope of Part B coverage extends. Be warned: A number of the services these practitioners provide are only narrowly or even minutely covered under Part B. For now, you just need to understand that it's possible for a wide range of institutions and practitioners to be involved in care covered by Part B.

One implication of the ongoing shift from inpatient to outpatient services is that you, as a Medicare beneficiary, will tend to pay more in premiums. This is because you get your Part A benefits based on taxes you paid as you worked, so you don't pay any extra for it as time goes on (unless you are one of the very few beneficiaries that purchases Part A). However, that is not true for Part B. You have to pay about 25 percent of the costs of this part of the Medicare program, and so when costs shift from Part A to Part B, you pay more of the Medicare burden in your monthly Part B premium compared to when Part

A paid for those services. In other words, the reason that your Part B premium almost always goes up every January is not only because of the increase in cost of medical services and the introduction of new and usually more expensive treatments, but also because of this inpatient to outpatient shift (that is, from Part A to premium Part B).

2. Assignment

Assignment means that a provider or physician consents to the following clauses when they give you a medical service or item:

- They agree to accept whatever Medicare says is the "approved amount" a provider may charge for his or her services. You, the beneficiary, will not be liable for any amount charged above that approved amount.

- They agree to receive the payment directly from Medicare; that is, they will not bill you for the full cost of the service.

- They agree to collect from you only the appropriate coinsurance and deductible and nothing more — they can do this right away or wait until the claim is processed.

Almost all institutional providers such as hospitals must take assignment.

Unless your state's laws dictate otherwise, most noninstitutional medical practitioners such as physicians and surgeons (even when part of a clinic) can choose to take payment in one of three ways with Medicare:

1. Noninstitutional medical practitioners can choose to "participate" in Medicare. For every calendar year they choose to participate, they must always accept Medicare assignment on every claim — that is, they will never charge you more

than the amount Medicare approves on a claim for a particular service. Generally, Medicare pays 80 percent of what it approves, while you pay 20 percent (your coinsurance). An exception to this rule is mental health therapy, which is currently split 50–50 with Medicare, although this policy is changing.

Note that the physicians may change their decision to participate in any given calendar year, but most who participate initally continue to do so in subsequent years.

There is another valuable benefit to going to a doctor that accepts assignment. If you happen to have a Medicare Supplement Policy (i.e., Medigap policy) that does not automatically get information from Medicare to pay its portion of a claim, it still must pay participating doctors directly.

The states that mandate that physicians always take assignment are Connecticut, Massachusetts, Minnesota, New York, Ohio, Pennsylvania, Rhode Island, and Vermont. If you live in one of these states, you don't have to worry about your doctor bills apart from your coinsurance. However, you still have to know the rules for those suppliers who are not physicians. These laws are governed by the state where the service is given, so if you live in Massachusetts and see a doctor in New Hampshire, this assignment regulation does not apply.

2. Noninstitutional medical practitioners can choose not to participate in assignment. On each Medicare service, nonparticipating practitioners have the option of taking assignment on each individual claim they file. For nonparticipating physicians and suppliers, Medicare's approved amount for what a practioner may charge for his or her services is always 5 percent less than what it would be for participating practitioners. Many physicians never take assignment.

If the practitioner chooses to take assignment on your claim, Medicare will usually pay 80 percent of the approved amount a practitioner may charge for his or her services, while you will pay 20 percent. The practitioner cannot charge you more than the amount approved by Medicare. If the practitioner doesn't take assignment on a claim, with the exception discussed in the next paragraph, he or she can charge you anything he or she wants, no matter what the approved amount is. In this case, you would generally be responsible for paying everything you were charged above 80 percent of the approved amount.

There is one important ceiling here. Under federal law, a physician cannot charge you more than what is called the *limiting charge*, which is the Medicare approved amount plus 15 percent. For example, suppose a surgeon not taking assignment does a procedure on you and submits a claim for $1,250. Medicare approves $1,000 (and pays $800), but you pay only $350 for the surgery. This is because you pay $200, that is, the 20 percent coinsurance of the Medicare-approved amount. But because the limiting charge is $1,150 ($1,000 plus 15 percent), you have to pay this $150 over the approved amount of $1,000 on top of the $200 coinsurance for a total of $350. This $150 is known as the excess charge; that is, the dollar difference between what Medicare approves and what the doctor can charge you. You, in effect, "save" $100 because the surgeon could only charge you $1,150 instead of the $1,250 he or she wanted to charge you. If the claim was for $1,100 and the approved amount was still $1,000, you would only be charged $300 for the surgery. The columns in Table 8 will help clarify this.

The second column shows what would happen if you go to a participating doctor for an office visit or get a walker from a participating equipment supply company. The column shows that Medicare approves the $100, pays the physician or supplier $80, and your coinsurance is the difference — $20.

The third column shows what happens if you go to a physician who does not participate regularly, but who decides to take assignment on your claim. He or she submits a charge for $115, but Medicare approves only $95, or 5 percent less than what it approves for the same thing from a physician participating in assignment. Because the doctor took assignment on this particular claim,

he or she cannot charge you $115; instead, he or she is stuck with the lower, approved amount of $95. Medicare will pay the physician 80 percent of the $95, which is $76, and you owe only $19 as your coinsurance.

In the fourth column, it is supposed that the physician doesn't take assignment. He or she submits a charge for $115 and Medicare approves the $95, which is the same as the nonparticipating physician that took assignment. Medicare will pay the same $76, but it will also show that the most the doctor can charge is $109.25, which is the limiting charge at 15 percent more than the $95 approved charge. You owe $33.25 (the $19.00 coinsurance plus the $14.25 excess charge).

If nonparticipating, non-physician suppliers and pharmacies take assignment, it would look just like the second column. In the fifth column it shows the costs if they don't take assignment. They are not bound by the limiting charge rule. If they charge $115, Medicare will approve $100 (the 5 percent reduction

TABLE 8
PART B PAYMENTS

	Participating Physician or Supplier Always Accepts Assignment	Nonparticipating Physician Accepts Assignment	Nonparticipating Physician Does Not Accept Assignment	Nonparticipating Supplier or Pharmacy Does Not Accept Assignment
Charge	$115.00	$115.00	$115.00	$115.00
Limiting Charge	N/A	N/A	$109.25	N/A
Approved	$100.00	$95.00	$95.00	$100.00
Medicare Pays	$80.00	$76.00	$76.00	$80.00
You Owe	$20.00	$19.00	$33.25	$35.00

applies only to nonparticipating physicians), it will pay $80, and you will be responsible for $35. If they charged $200, you would be responsible for $120 because there is no limiting charge!

It will be helpful for you to remember that the limiting charge does not apply to the following:

- Durable medical equipment
- Vaccinations
- Orthotics and prosthetics
- Surgical dressings

A physician or practitioner that does not take assignment on a claim can charge you up front for his or her service. You may be asked to pay for the service while in his or her office. The practitioner has to submit your claim to Medicare and Medicare will send you the check. Medicare will also send you a Medicare Summary Notice (MSN) at once, so you won't have to wait the usual three months that Medicare waits to send you these notices to figure out what happened on your claim.

3. There is the very rare situation in which a physician chooses to opt out or exclude himself or herself from the Medicare program. Basically, the physician refuses to take any payments from Medicare. The physician has to tell you up front that any service he or she gives you cannot be billed to Medicare and you will be responsible for all the costs. In other words, the physician can charge you whatever he or she wants. Only a very small handful of physicians (less than 1 percent) have done this.

If, in an extremely rare situation, a doctor asks you to sign a private contract with him or her (this is how he or she opts out of Medicare), and you do so, you will be fully responsible for the doctor's entire bill, no matter what it is. Your Medigap will not help, and your other insurance policies — especially if they are secondary to your Medicare — likely won't pay anything.

Obviously your strategy should be that if you get services in a state that does not mandate assignment, try to use a participating physician in order to manage your medical costs better. Never go to a supplier such as a durable medical equipment supplier that does not take assignment on all of your claims — you can get charged any fee if you do this.

Be aware, if you are in Original Medicare, that all Medigap policies will pay the Part B coinsurance amounts (the 20 percent you normally pay). Some policies will pay the excess charge, that is, the 15 percent extra that physicians can charge on non-assigned claims.

The following are some additional rules about assignment:

- If a doctor does a lab test in his or her office, the doctor must always accept assignment on the test.
- If you have both Medicare and Medicaid, a doctor, supplier, or pharmacy must always accept assignment on your claim. They must also accept assignment if you are a Qualified Medicare Beneficiary.
- If you get a Medicare Part B covered drug from an enrolled supplier or pharmacy, the supplier must take assignment on the drug claim.
- As part of the assigned versus non-assigned issue, you should know that on

any assigned claim, a physician or supplier can't ask you to pay up front and in full for the service. They can ask you to pay up front for whatever Medicare won't pay, which includes the amount of the deductible you have not yet satisfied that calendar year and the coinsurance or co-payment for the service or item.

- Physicians are not required to treat Medicare beneficiaries; they can decide on a person-by-person basis or on a service-by-service basis whom to treat. Just because a physician participates in Medicare, this does not mean that he or she has to take you as a patient or even see you if you want a service from him or her.

3. Filing Claims

You will almost never have to personally file a Medicare claim. All Medicare certified institutional providers must do this as part of their agreement with the federal government to serve as a Medicare provider. Also, all physicians and practitioners must file for you whether or not they are participating providers (that is, always take assignment), even if they are not participating and they do not take assignment on your claim. (See section 2. for more on assignment). In the remote situation that a physician who has disavowed Medicare renders an emergency service to you, he or she has to bill Medicare.

All participating suppliers and pharmacies must also file for you. If they don't participate, they must file for you if they take assignment on a particular claim. Nonparticipating pharmacies must do so too, because they must take assignment on the few drugs covered under Part B.

You might have to file a claim under Part B when a supplier or pharmacy is not participating, does not take assignment on your claim, and refuses to file for you. The exception is that only a supplier can file a claim for diabetes testing items and supplies.

You may be asking, if all Part B drugs must be assigned, why aren't pharmacies forced to take assignment? It's because they can also sell you supplies and durable medical equipment; they don't have to take assignment on these things. You should understand that if a durable medical equipment supplier sells you a covered Part B drug that is given to you via equipment such as a nebulizer, they also have to be registered as a pharmacy to dispense that drug.

Finally, there are time limits on filing. Generally, a Medicare claim must be filed by the end of the calendar year after the year in which the services were provided. For example, if you get a piece of medical equipment on February 22, 2010, the Medicare claim for that item must be filed by December 31, 2011.

In the extremely rare circumstance that you have to file a claim but you miss the end of the "calendar year after the year" rule, you still have the right to file the claim and ask that the time limit be waived. If you come up with a good excuse, you may get your claim approved. However, if your claim is denied, you have all the appeal rights discussed in the Chapter 14 to contest this. And, if you don't appeal, you are responsible for the whole sum.

If a provider was supposed to file for you and was not timely in so doing, it generally can't charge you for the services it rendered (except what you would have had to pay if it had filed on time, i.e., the coinsurance).

Finally, the Medicare program is subject to federal law which requires it to pay claims on a timely basis. When a Medicare Administrative Contractor gets a claim with all the information needed to approve it, the contractor has to process it in 30 calendar days. If the contractor doesn't process it within the time limit, Medicare has to pay interest on the claim. You may see on your Medicare Summary Notice that your provider received interest or, in the case that you are due the money when the claim was delayed in processing, you get the interest. If it was not processed within 30 days and you do not receive interest, contact Medicare.

4. Waiver of Liability: Advanced Beneficiary Notice

One requirement for any non-preventative medical service or supply is that it has to be medically reasonable and necessary in order for Medicare to pay for it. This means that the diagnostic or curative procedures given to you must, according to prevailing medical standards and practices, be appropriate for your condition(s) or diagnoses. Under Medicare law, this medical necessity test must always be met before Medicare pays a claim.

There is a protection given to Medicare beneficiaries under this law: You cannot be held liable for the cost of a procedure that Medicare determines was not medically necessary. This is because the law presumes that you, as a layperson, could not know that a particular service was not medically necessary. It further presumes that the practitioner should know that it was not necessary. If Medicare denies a claim as not medically necessary — it doesn't matter if it was assigned or unassigned — the physician or practitioner cannot charge you for the service. This is called the *waiver of liability* because you are not liable for the cost of the service.

There are some exceptions. One is that if you had a similar condition and received a similar service that was then denied as not medically necessary, the law now presumes that you should know that the service is not medically necessary, and the waiver of liability will not apply. A simple example might be that you have a condition that you feel a physician's check-up is needed every month, but Medicare has denied such a claim as it believes a check-up every three months is appropriate, and that a once-a-month frequency is not medically necessary. As you have received a notice to this effect, you would be liable for visits exceeding the quarterly frequency.

Another exception is the Advanced Beneficiary Notice. If your doctor or practitioner believes that the service he or she is going to give you, or that you ask for, is not or is probably not medically necessary, the physician will insist you sign an Advanced Beneficiary Notice. This form will list the specific service or procedure involved and state why your doctor or practitioner thinks it is not medically necessary. This will make you liable for the cost of the procedure, and he or she may charge you any fee he or she wishes, as long as he or she states what it will be. This process is in place to protect the doctor or practitioner from getting stuck with the cost. If this happens, you will in all likelihood have to pay for it because your Medigap policy will not pay for it, and if you have any other insurance policy, it probably will not pay either if Medicare does not.

If you go ahead with the procedure, you can insist that a claim be filed anyway. This is called a *demand claim* or a *demand bill*. Medicare will look at the claim and decide if the service was medically necessary. If it decides it was, Medicare will pay its share and it will impose the approved amount (if the doctor participates or took assignment) or the limiting charge (if the doctor did not accept assignment). If an expensive fee was charged up front, it will be reduced. There is no downside to asking for this demand claim to be filed.

Note that this Advance Beneficiary Notice routine applies only for medical necessity issues. It does not apply for services that are simply not covered by Medicare. For example, if you go to a dermatologist for Botox for your wrinkles, the physician can charge you any price as this is a cosmetic procedure and is, by Medicare law, never covered. The physician also does not have to give you the Advance Beneficiary Notice in this case.

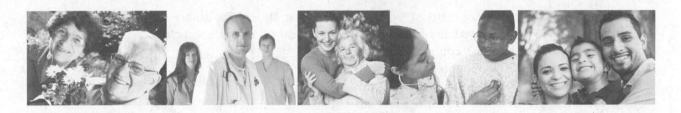

4

Part B: Details of Coverage

This chapter gives you details about Part B coverage of practitioners, services, and items. Chapter 5 will discuss the Part B coverage of durable medical equipment.

1. The Most Commonly Covered Part B Services

The following are the major categories (in terms of payments) of diagnostic and therapeutic services that Medicare will cover under Part B. These are services that anyone might need and therefore you will want to have some understanding of. You should assume that each service discussed is subject to both the annual deductible and the 20 percent coinsurance; if there are exceptions to this general rule, they will be noted.

You will receive from Medicare a handbook called *Medicare & You*, which provides an extensive list of what Part B covers. This chapter will go through the services in terms of what you will most frequently use with the idea that the more you use it, the more you will want to know about it.

For all the services listed, remember that each is subject to the yearly deductible (which is $155 in 2010), coinsurance, or co-payment unless otherwise stated. You should also presume that the limiting charge applies unless explicitly said otherwise. Sometimes under Medicare, a particular service must be assigned or even a particular type of practitioner must take assignment on a claim. (For more details on assignment and limiting charges, see section **2.** in Chapter 3.) Where assignment applies to a practice or service, it will be stated.

It should be made very clear that Medigap policies must pay the coinsurance or co-payment as determined by the Medicare Administrative Contractor, sometimes still known as a carrier. While coinsurance usually amounts to 20 percent of the total cost of the service, it is 50 percent for most psychiatric services, and it varies from 20 percent to 40 percent for hospital outpatient services. Certain services even have different, specified percentages. Your Medigap policy has to pay the coinsurance amount no matter what the percentage is. Of course, the catastrophic policies only pay part of whatever the coinsurance or co-payment is. In other words, policy K pays half the coinsurance, and L pays three-quarters. See Chapter 10, section **2.10** for the details. (Note: This policy of payment may not apply to some very old Medigap policies originally purchased many years ago.)

The following sections cover the vast majority of all Part B services.

1.1 Doctors' services

Just about any type of diagnostic or therapeutic service performed by a doctor is covered by Medicare, including any visits you make to a doctor's office and any visits a doctor makes to you in the hospital, a nursing facility, or in your own home. You should understand that if you are in a non-Medicare facility (e.g., assisted living facility), or even if you are in a Medicare-certified facility but your stay there is not covered by Medicare (e.g., you are in a Skilled Nursing Facility but you ran out of covered days), the doctor's visit is still covered if medically necessary.

The term "doctor" here refers to general and family practitioners and also specialists and sub-specialists of all kinds including surgeons, radiologists, pathologists, and hematologists: essentially, any of those with a Doctor of Medicine (MD) or Doctor of Osteopathic Medicine (DO) degree. If medically appropriate, Medicare may cover the services of consulting physicians your primary physician brings in to help with a tough case.

Medicare Part B also covers necessary supplies the doctor may use in treating you, such as splints and dressings. Most drugs you receive in the doctor's office as part of your treatment are covered.

Medicare will also pay certain other medical practitioners in the same way (but not always the same amount) as doctors even though they do not all have a doctorate-level degree. These medical practitioners include:

- Anesthesiologist's assistants
- Certified nurse midwives
- Clinical psychologists
- Clinical social workers
- Certified registered nurse anesthetists
- Nurse practitioners
- Clinical nurse specialists
- Physician assistants

These medical practitioners must meet both state and federal requirements for their individual practices; these often include one level or another of supervision by a physician. Medicare will cover only those services which are recognized by state regulations as being within the appropriate scope of practice. As these regulations vary considerably, it is impossible to spell all this out in detail, but these individual practitioners know the rules for their particular states quite well. Note that the practitioners listed above must take assignments on claims.

1.2 Radiology procedures

Radiology procedures, whether diagnostic or curative, are covered. Typically, two bills will be issued to you: one for the actual X-ray, MRI, or CAT scan, and another for the radiologist who interprets the test for your doctor or surgeon. Radiation therapy procedures are subject to the limiting charge.

1.3 Diagnostic tests

A large variety of diagnostic tests are covered, including electrocardiography (EKG), electroencephalography (EEG), spinal tap, cystoscopy, and endoscopies. As with radiology, you may see two charges made to you: one for the test itself, and another from the doctor who interprets it.

Note that diagnostic tests are subject to the limiting charge.

1.4 Lab tests

Lab tests particular to laboratory operation, also known as *clinical laboratory tests*, include urinalysis, blood tests, and stool culture tests. While many doctors' offices perform some of the simpler tests, these tests are often more complex. Medicare pays for these tests in full with no deductible or coinsurance charges to you. Labs and doctors' offices must take assignment on these claims.

1.5 Hospital outpatient departments and clinics

Part B covers the extremely wide range of diagnostic and therapeutic services rendered to you in a hospital as an outpatient. These services include same-day surgery, lab tests, X-rays and other diagnostic tests, radiation treatment, chemo, splints, casts, and mental health therapy. As with any hospital service, the hospital must take assignment for these services.

These services are paid under an outpatient prospective payment system, so instead of the straight 20 percent coinsurance, you will pay a co-payment. However, be warned that your actual co-payment amount may be more than 20 percent of the Medicare allowance. In some cases, it can be as high as 40 percent.

You should also know that for any given procedure paid under this system, your co-payment can never exceed that year's inpatient deductible ($1,100 in 2010). Most Medicare beneficiaries are not affected by this exception to the general rule because all Medigap policies and most third-party insurance pays for the whole co-payment.

You will also be separately billed by the physicians you see and possibly by some you do not see (e.g., pathologist or radiologist). The rules discussed in Chapter 3, section 2. (Assignment) govern the payment of these physicians' bills.

1.6 Emergency rooms

Diagnostic and therapeutic services rendered to you in the emergency room are covered under Part B. As emergency rooms are part of a hospital, these services are paid under the outpatient prospective payment system discussed in section 1.5, and the hospital has to take assignment.

Remember that if you are admitted to the same hospital within three days for the same condition that required diagnostic tests in the emergency room (or the outpatient department or clinic), the charges for those emergency room services will be folded into your inpatient bill.

Warning: One of the big differences between Original Medicare and Medicare Advantage (Part C) is the use of emergency rooms. Generally, Medicare Advantage heavily discourages the use of emergency rooms for any but the most dire of circumstances, so follow your Medicare Advantage's managed care organization or health plan's rules as very best you can for this type of care. (Chapter 9 discusses your rights to get emergency or urgently needed care.)

1.7 Home health visits

If you have both Part A and B of Medicare, home health visits are automatically covered under Part A or Part B.

If you only have Part B, you always qualify for this benefit (as long as you meet the other requirements listed in Chapter 2, section 3., on home health care, such as being homebound). You do not have to pay an annual deductible or coinsurance — Medicare pays 100 percent. The exception occurs if you get durable medical equipment or supplies through your home health agency. For these, the usual Part

B deductible and coinsurance rules apply. This goes for osteoporosis drugs as well (see section **2.21** for more information about drugs covered under Part B). Note that home health agencies always have to take assignment.

1.8 Therapy

Physical therapy, speech-language pathology, and occupational therapy are vitally important to Medicare beneficiaries and can be delivered by a wide variety of providers. In Chapter 2 it was discussed that you can get these services under Part A as a hospital or Skilled Nursing Facility inpatient, or when you are under the care of a home health agency (whether under Part A or B). However, you can also get the services as an outpatient under Part B in a hospital outpatient department or clinic (in which case you pay a co-payment). You can also get these services in a Comprehensive Outpatient Rehabilitation Facility (see section **1.11** for more information), or from a rehabilitation agency, or in a doctor's office. In all these cases the 20 percent coinsurance applies.

Medicare covers the services given by independent physical therapists, speech-language pathologists, and occupational therapists. Independent physical therapists, speech-language pathologists, and occupational therapists can choose to participate in assignment, or not, just like doctors. Be sure to find out if they are participating and whether they will take assignment in your particular case. Even if they do not take assignment, they are subject to the limiting charge.

These therapies must be considered rehabilitative, not treatment to maintain a certain state, and must be given under a plan of care certified by a physician. These services can be rendered in the therapist's office, in the patient's home, or in some other settings. To receive the services in the home, the patient does not need to be homebound, and no additional payment is made for the therapists to travel to a home. Note that part of the actual therapy may be given by therapy assistants. Physical therapy includes not only the more traditional movement therapies, but can also include special heat, light, bath, and ultrasound therapies.

Before you get too comfortable with this particular benefit, you should know that each year or so legislation may impose outpatient therapy caps on how much Medicare will pay for therapy services for you in a calendar year. Specifically, legislation exists that automatically imposes financial limitations on the dollar amount Medicare will pay for most outpatient therapy services. This dollar amount, or cap is applied to physical therapy and speech-language pathology added together, and separately to occupational therapy. The limit or cap in 2010 is $1,860. This means that in 2010, Medicare paid for a total of $1,860 per patient for all the outpatient physical therapy and speech-language pathology, and up to the same dollar amount for all the outpatient occupational therapy.

There was an exception to the caps in 2009. If you exceeded the caps and the therapist attested that the services were medically necessary and documentation existed in your medical record to this effect, as all non-screening Medicare services have to be medically necessary, this justified genuinely needed therapy. Medicare paid for these services even though the cap was exceeded. This exception may or may not apply in future years.

You should know that no matter what the situation is in a given calendar year, there exist some exceptions to the caps that are always in place. For one, if your physical therapy is given in a hospital outpatient department or emergency room, the cap never applies. If you get your services under Part A as an inpatient in a hospital or a Skilled Nursing Facility, the caps do not apply.

Finally, if your therapy is part of your covered home health agency episode of care, the cap does not apply, whether or not Part A or Part B is paying for your episode. You should keep these exceptions in mind, especially the hospital outpatient one, in case the caps are put in place in a future year without the generous exceptions in place in 2009. Thus if the caps are in place, but you go (for example) to a hospital outpatient department for therapy, they won't apply.

1.9 Ambulance

Medicare covers ambulance services, but will only pay for transportation to four places:

- Hospital
- Skilled Nursing Facility
- End-stage renal dialysis facility
- Your home (Note: If you go from your home to your doctor's office, this is not covered.)

Medicare will pay for your emergency ambulance transportation (e.g., after a heart attack). It may pay for your transport to one of these places in nonemergency situations, but there are several conditions. One is that your doctor must certify that your medical condition is such that transportation by ambulance is necessary. Another is that the use of another form of transport would be detrimental to your health; for example, suppose you were unconscious, bleeding badly, could be moved only by stretcher, or were bed-confined. Note that being confined to a wheelchair is not considered necessary to be transported by ambulance; that is, just because you are wheelchair-bound does not mean you qualify for ambulance transport.

In all cases, Medicare will pay for transport by ambulance only to the nearest appropriate facility. If you demand to be transported to a hospital in another community because you recently moved from there and are familiar with its hospital, Medicare would pay only what it would have paid to take you to your new community's hospital.

Medicare does cover air (e.g., airplane and helicopter) ambulance services, where accessibility, remoteness, or the need for more speed than ground ambulance can provide deems air transport necessary.

All ambulance services are required to take assignment on Medicare claims.

1.10 Pathology

Many pathology services have a professional component in which a physician, usually a pathologist, views a specimen or slide and renders a medical opinion. This professional component is billed and payable by the beneficiary at the usual 20 percent coinsurance.

1.11 Comprehensive Outpatient Rehabilitation Facilities (CORF)

Comprehensive Outpatient Rehabilitation Facilities (CORF) provide a wide range of comprehensive, coordinated rehabilitative therapy services and related treatments that are covered by Part B. Some of these facilities are stand-alone, while others are associated with hospitals.

To receive covered services, you must be under the care of a physician who certifies that you need skilled rehabilitative services, and the facility must develop a detailed plan of treatment for your rehabilitation. You have the right to participate in formulating your plan. While a CORF can give quite a wide variety of services, it centers around physical therapy, speech-language pathology, occupational and respiratory therapy, and includes social and psychological and some nursing services, as well as the provision of prosthetic and orthotic devices. Typically, these services are given in the facility, but it may provide certain therapy services at other locations (e.g., nursing home).

As part of this benefit, you may be able to have a physical or an occupational therapist visit your home to assess whether or not your home environment might be adverse to your recovery under your plan, and the therapist may make recommendations to improve your home environment. However, while Medicare will pay for this single home evaluation visit, Medicare will not pay the cost of, for example, replacing slippery tile with a nonskid surface.

CORFs must always accept assignment on Medicare claims. Also note that a CORF cannot end your treatment unless it notifies you in writing that it intends to do so, and reminds you of the special rights you have to appeal this before it is done.

1.12 Mental health services

Medicare covers visits to physicians, psychiatrists, clinical psychologists, and clinical social workers. It will pay for a wide variety of mental health services including diagnostic and laboratory tests to help diagnose your condition and to determine if treatments are helping you. It also covers therapeutic services such as individual and group therapy, some limited counseling with family members so they can assist with your treatment, therapy activities such as occupational therapy to improve your condition, and drugs administered by a physician. (If you have Part D, it will cover prescription drugs.)

Under some circumstances, Medicare may also cover a special intensive outpatient mental health therapy regime called Partial Hospitalization. This approach is designed to keep beneficiaries out of hospital inpatient psychiatric care and in a community setting. See section **2.32** for details.

Medicare doesn't cover support groups, job skill assessments, or meals eaten during a course of treatment.

1.12a Special payment rules

The Part B "outpatient mental health limitation" must be clearly understood. (This information does not apply to inpatient services; there are special, separate limitations there.) This limitation does not apply to diagnostic services (i.e., testing for and the evaluation of a mental illness), or to see how you have responded to treatment, or to see if your treatment should be changed. Rather, it applies to the therapy itself. The limitation is that Medicare has paid a smaller percentage of its approved amount, not 80 percent as is the norm for Part B services. You will therefore end up paying half of all the approved charges.

The good news is that beginning in 2010, the percentage will gradually increase so that it will be 80 percent by 2014. In a few years, Part B will pay the usual 80 percent of your approved amount, just like most Part B services. The phase-ins are as follows:

- 2009: 50 percent
- 2010–2011: 55 percent (phase-in begins)
- 2012: 60 percent
- 2013: 65 percent
- 2014: 80 percent (phase-in complete)

You need an explanation of how this limitation works, because, confusingly, some Medicare information discusses this unique limitation in two parts. It tells you that through 2009 it takes the usual approved charge for the service and multiplies this by 62.5 percent, and then multiplies this by 80 percent, which, if you do the math, is the same as multiplying the original approved amount by 50 percent. Why does

Medicare befuddle you this way? It's only because the annual Part B deductible ($135 in 2009, $155 in 2010) has to be subtracted after the first calculation and before the second, which can result in a small difference in what Medicare pays and what you are liable for. However, if you have already satisfied your deductible, your liability will be half or 50 percent of the Medicare approved amount rather than 80 percent.

It may help to show a complete example of how this limitation works. For example, suppose you incur a mental condition and, after an evaluation visit that satisfies all but $50 of your annual Part B deductible, you have ten psychotherapy sessions on which your psychiatrist takes assignment and charges the Medicare approved amount of $150 each. Your liability is figured as follows:

- Total allowed amount = 10 (visits) x $150 (per visit) = $1,500

- $1,500 x 62.5% = $937.50 (the limitation)

- Subtract your remaining Part B deductible: $937.50 - $50 (remaining deductible) = $887.50

- Apply the usual 80% coinsurance to this: $887.50 x 80% = $710

- $1,500 - $710 (Medicare pays) = $790 (your liability)

1.13 Ambulatory surgical centers

Ambulatory surgical centers are outpatient facilities in which a wide variety of medical procedures are performed. Three general requirements must be met for Medicare to pay for care in these centers:

- Your procedure should not be done in one of these centers if it is expected that you will subsequently be hospitalized.

- Your procedure should take no more than 90 minutes.

- Your recovery time should not exceed four hours.

Deductible and coinsurance both apply. Ambulatory surgical centers are paid on a set fee schedule. Remember that the surgeon's fee is not included in the payment to the center; you will get a separate bill for that, which Medicare will cover at the usual 80 percent of the approved amount. These centers do not have to accept assignment, but are subject to the limiting charge. If your ambulatory surgical center is part of a hospital, it is paid on the same set fee schedule and you pay the coinsurance, and not a hospital outpatient co-payment, which can be more expensive.

2. Information about Coverage for Other Services

This section gives you detailed information on the many other kinds of services that Medicare may or may not cover. Preventative services are also included because sometimes the same service is covered as preventative and sometimes as diagnostic. And, unless otherwise noted, all these Part B services are subject to the annual Part B deductible ($155 in 2010) and the usual 20 percent coinsurance.

2.1 Abdominal aortic screening

Medicare beneficiaries at risk for an abdominal aortic aneurysm can be referred for an ultrasound screening test, but only as part of their "Welcome to Medicare" physical exam, which is discussed in section 2.45. That is, you'll typically get a referral from your examining physician to have this ultrasound done. The annual deductible does not apply to this ultrasound.

Here, *at risk* means that you have a family history of aortic aneurysm, or that you are a man 65 to 75 who has smoked at least 100 cigarettes in your lifetime.

2.2 Abortion

Medicare does cover abortion, but only when the life of the mother is endangered, or rape or incest has occurred.

2.3 Acupuncture

Acupuncture is not covered by Medicare.

2.4 Alcoholism

Treatment for alcoholism is covered under Part B, but it is subject to the mental health limitation discussed in section **1.12**. Covered treatments include drug therapy, psychotherapy, patient education, and possibly limited family counseling. Coverage extends to chemical aversion therapy, but not electrical aversion therapy.

Part A will cover inpatient stays for detoxification and also for rehabilitation, but only when this has proven unsuccessful on an outpatient basis, or the beneficiary has another condition which, along with the rehab process, might warrant this level of care. Part D covers some anti-alcoholism drugs.

2.5 Anesthesia

Medicare pays for the services of anesthesiologists, as well as, where recognized by state law, those of certified registered nurse anesthetists (CRNAs) and anesthesiologist assistants.

2.6 Artificial hearts

Artificial hearts are covered under Medicare when two criteria are met. One is if the device that is implanted is part of a study that the Food and Drug Administration (FDA) has approved; the other is if certain Centers for Medicare & Medicaid Services (CMS) clinical research criteria are met. The surgical team that performs the operation can tell you if these requirements are met. While you need Part A to cover your hospital stay, Part B will cover the surgeon's fees and other involved Part B services.

2.7 Blood

Medicare will pay for whole blood or packed blood cells under Part B, but there is a special Medicare blood deductible of three pints per calendar year. That is, you pay in full for the first three pints, and Medicare will pay for 80 percent of each subsequent pint required.

Note that this once-per-calendar-year, three-pint deductible applies whether Part A or Part B is involved. As mentioned in Chapter 2, if you get blood while you are a Part A inpatient, Part A pays the whole cost after the blood deductible is satisfied, not just 80 percent.

You are encouraged to donate blood for yourself in advance or to have others donate in your name, as any pint donated releases you from paying for any of the first three deductible pints. Similarly, if the provider gets the blood from a blood bank at no charge, it cannot make you pay for it.

2.8 Bone mass measurement

The bone mass measurement screening test (sometimes called a bone mineral density or BMD study) is available for those at risk for osteoporosis. *At risk* in this case refers to women who are being treated for low levels of estrogen and who are at risk for osteoporosis based on medical history.

Women and men alike may be considered at risk if any of the following four conditions are met:

- Your X-rays show possible osteoporosis, osteopenia, or vertebrae fractures.
- You are on (or are planning to begin) prednisone or steroid-type drug treatment.

- You have hyperparathyroidism.
- You are being monitored to see if you osteoporosis drug treatment is working.

If any of the at-risk situations apply to you, you qualify to get this test every two years (23 months must have passed since your last test), or more often if it is medically necessary. These tests are usually done with X-rays.

2.9 Cardiac rehabilitation programs

Medicare covers cardiac rehabilitation programs, which typically include exercise, education, and counseling for those beneficiaries who have significant heart disease. This includes those who have —

- had a heart attack in the last 12 months,
- had coronary bypass surgery,
- stable angina pectoris,
- had a heart valve repair or replacement,
- had angioplasty or coronary stenting, or
- had a heart or heart-lung transplant.

Medicare will pay its share for up to 36 sessions (usually two or three sessions a week) and possibly more, depending on medical circumstances. Sometimes these sessions are given by a hospital outpatient clinic or department, and sometimes in physician clinics.

People with congestive heart failure are not covered.

2.10 Cardiovascular disease screening

To help prevent heart attacks and strokes, Medicare covers a screening blood test for your cholesterol, lipid, and triglyceride levels once every five years. As with any clinical lab test, no coinsurance or deductible applies. Note that Medicare covers the cost of the test, but your visit to the doctor to review the test results is subject to the usual deductible and coinsurance.

2.11 Chemotherapy

Medicare covers chemotherapy. It pays for all Food and Drug Administration (FDA) approved on-label use of chemotherapeutic agents as well as off-label use when the application is recognized as appropriate. On-label use means using a drug to treat a condition that the FDA has specifically approved for the drug, while off-label use is treating a condition not specifically approved by the FDA for that particular drug. Medicare Administrative Contractors sometimes approve local coverage policies for other off-label use.

Remember that while most chemotherapy is given in a provider or physician setting, such as a hospital outpatient clinic or doctor's office, some chemotherapy drugs that can be prescribed for use in the home qualify for Part B payment. See section **2.21** for information about this exception where Part B will pay for prescription drugs.

2.12 Chiropractic

Only one service by a chiropractor is covered under Part B, which is a manual manipulation of the spine to correct a subluxation when a spinal bone is out of position. If your chiropractor takes an X-ray to help diagnose your back problem, the X-ray is not covered because only the manual manipulation is covered. As a chiropractor is considered a physician for this one service covered by Part B, the limiting charge applies.

2.13 Clinical trials and research studies

In a huge exception to Medicare's general policy not to pay for items or services that have not shown themselves to be effective, Medicare will help with the costs of certain experimental treatments. This is good for Medicare patients because, if they are allowed to participate in one of the qualified clinical trials that Medicare has accepted, Medicare will pay for the routine care they receive in the trial.

More specifically, Medicare won't pay for the specific item, drug, or protocol that is being evaluated in the trial, or for any data collection, for clinical or diagnostic tests solely related to data requirements (e.g., the protocol may call for a monthly X-ray which Medicare wouldn't usually cover), or for anything that is typically provided free-of-charge by the trial sponsor. Medicare will not pay for something on a trial basis that it would not cover outside of a trial situation. For example, Medicare would in all likelihood not cover a cosmetic procedure or a preventative service.

Medicare will pay for routine care including all conventional care, and also for the implementation of the investigational agent, device, or drug (e.g., if the trial involves a chemo drug that has to be infused, Medicare will help pay for the infusion procedure, but not for the drug itself). Medicare will also help pay for the care needed to clinically monitor you and the effect of the device on your condition. Importantly, it covers care you need to prevent or to deal with complications caused by the new approach. It's especially helpful to know that Medicare will cover complications.

Medicare doesn't approve these trials on a case-by-case basis. Rather, trials conducted by the federal agencies that typically conduct these (e.g., National Institutes of Health and Veterans Health Administration) and groups directly sponsored by these agencies automatically qualify. Also, trials conducted under an investigational new drug application the Food and Drug Administration has reviewed are covered. Other principal investigators can self-certify that their trials met the criteria set by Medicare, and thus achieve qualification.

One important twist to this Medicare coverage is that even Medicare Advantage managed care organizations and health plans that have strict rules about the use of in-network providers must make these trials available to their Medicare members, even though they use out-of-network providers. This is because Medicare beneficiaries in managed care always have coverage of what is available to those who are in Original Medicare, and so they must be covered here even though these trials will almost always be made available by nonnetwork providers. If you are not in Medicare Advantage, but have a Medicare Supplement or Medigap policy, it will pay its share of what Medicare covers in these trials.

At any given point in time there are thousands of trials being planned or taking place. The best places for information are on the Web. The Resources file on the CD includes links to trials.

Be extremely careful; be sure that you fully understand the trial before you agree to sign the informed consent to participate in the trial.

2.14 Colorectal cancer screening

Medicare covers a number of different tests for colorectal cancer screening. These tests help detect colorectal cancer and precancerous growths to promote early treatment.

Any Medicare beneficiary age 50 or older can get a fecal occult blood test, and can do so every 12 months under Part B's coverage. As it's a lab test, deductible and coinsurance don't apply. The test has to be ordered by a physician.

You have to determine if you are at high risk for this type of cancer. In this case, it specifically means that one or more of the following apply to you:

- You have, or a close relative has, had colorectal cancer or an adenomatous polyp (the type of polyp which could be cancerous).

- You have a family history of familial adenomatous polyposis (multiple adenomatous polyps).

- You have a family history of hereditary non-polyposis colorectal cancer.

- You have inflammatory bowel disease, Crohn's disease, or inflammatory ulcerative colitis.

There are three different tests involved (i.e., flexible sigmoidoscopy, colonoscopy, and barium enema), and four different disease threat levels (i.e., 50 or older, younger than 50, high risk, and normal risk). See Table 9 for a breakdown of this information.

For those 50 or older and not at high risk, in addition to the fecal occult blood test every year, one of the following invasive tests is covered every 48 months (four years) or 120 months (ten years):

- You are covered for a colonoscopy, and you can get one every 120 months. The exception is if you had a flexible sigmoidoscopy, you can have a colonoscopy covered only 48 months after that flexible sigmoidoscopy.

- You can get a flexible sigmoidoscopy every 48 months. The exception is if you had a colonoscopy, you can have a covered flexible sigmoidoscopy only 48 months after that colonoscopy.

- You can get a barium enema every 48 months.

For those 50 or older who are at high risk, in addition to the fecal occult blood test every year, one of the following invasive tests is covered every 24 months (two years) or 48 months (four years):

- You are covered for a colonoscopy every 24 months.

- You can get a flexible sigmoidoscopy every 48 months.

- You can get a barium enema every 24 months.

For those younger than 50 and not at high risk, only one test is covered, which is the colonoscopy, and you can get one every 120 months.

TABLE 9
COLORECTAL SCREENING TESTS

Test	50 or Older Normal Risk	50 or Older High Risk	Younger than 50 Normal Risk	Younger than 50 High Risk
Fecal occult blood	Every 12 months	Every 12 months	Not covered	Not covered
Colonoscopy	Every 120 months*	Every 24 months	Every 120 months	Every 24 months
Barium enema**	Every 48 months	Every 24 months	Not covered	Every 24 months
Flexible sigmoidoscopy	Every 48 months***	Every 48 months	Not covered	Every 24 months

* Exception: You have to wait four years after you get a screening flexible sigmoidoscopy to qualify for this test.
** The barium enema is given instead of a flexible sigmoidoscopy or a colonoscopy.
*** Exception: You have to wait ten years after you get a colonoscopy to qualify for this test.

For those younger than 50 who are at high risk, one of the following invasive tests is covered every 24 months (two years):

- You can get a colonoscopy every 24 months.
- You can get a barium enema every 24 months.

The deductible does not apply to any of these colorectal cancer-screening tests.

If for some reason you get a flexible sigmoidoscopy or a colonoscopy as a hospital outpatient, you pay a 25 percent coinsurance rate.

2.15 Community Mental Health Centers (CMHCs)

Community Mental Health Centers (CMHCs) are entities that fall under the Public Health Service laws, but which can obtain Medicare participation approval to furnish one service in particular: partial hospitalization, which is an intensive mental health service. You should make sure your center has the participation approval if you go into its partial hospitalization program.

Partial hospitalization services must be given on an assigned basis under Medicare. It is also possible for you to get covered mental health services at one of the CMHCs if it is a clinic, for example, if you get individual psychotherapy from a doctor there. As the physician may or may not participate, the usual rules for physician Part B services would apply.

2.16 Cosmetic procedures

Medicare never covers cosmetic surgery procedures or surgery to enhance your looks. However, if you have suffered an injury, or if you need to improve the function of a malformation of a limb or body part, these procedures are covered. Medicare specifically covers breast reconstruction after a mastectomy for breast cancer.

2.17 Dentistry

Dentistry is not covered, and any service dealing with the filling, extraction, or treatment of teeth or the preparation of the jaw for dentures is not covered. These are not even covered if the work has to be done in a hospital, such as the removal of an impacted tooth, but, oddly, the hospital stay itself would be covered if the procedure was medically necessary.

An exception to this general noncoverage of dental services is that if dental work is specifically needed to prepare a patient for another, covered service (e.g., the removal of a tooth so therapeutic radiation can be given), this is covered, even when this work is done by a dentist. In these very rare cases, the dentist is considered a physician and the limiting charge rule applies.

2.18 Diabetes screenings

Medicare covers screenings for diabetes for those beneficiaries who are at risk for this disease. You have to have at least one of the following four risk factors:

- High blood pressure
- Dyslipidemia (i.e., history of abnormal cholesterol and triglyceride levels)
- History of high blood sugar
- Obesity

Or at least two of the following four risk factors:

- You are age 65 or older.
- You are overweight.
- You have a family history of diabetes (i.e., a parent or sibling had or has it).
- You had gestational diabetes (i.e., diabetes during pregnancy) or had a baby weighing more than nine pounds.

You get one screening a year if you were never previously tested or, if you were, and you were not diagnosed with pre-diabetes. If you have been diagnosed with pre-diabetes, you get two screenings a year (not closer than six months apart). The screening test is a lab test of your blood for elevated blood glucose. The specific tests that are covered are a fasting blood glucose test, and one of two kinds of post glucose challenge tests. As with any lab test, deductible and coinsurance do not apply.

2.18a Diabetes self-management training

Medicare will cover diabetes self-management training under the following three conditions:

- You have diabetes and you become a Medicare beneficiary.

- You have been a Medicare beneficiary, but are now diagnosed with diabetes.

- You are at risk for complications from diabetes. This covers the following conditions:

  * You have difficulty controlling your blood sugar.

  * You begin taking diabetes medication or you switch from oral diabetes medication to insulin.

  * You are diagnosed with an eye disease related to diabetes.

  * You have foot problems, including a lack of sensation, ulcers, deformities, or you suffered an amputation.

  * You have been to the emergency room, or you were admitted to a hospital, because of diabetes.

  * You have kidney disease related to diabetes.

Medicare specifically approves of the diabetes self-management training program. Your doctor or other health-care provider (e.g.,

nurse practitioner or physician assistant) must provide a prescription or written order for you to have this service, and a plan of care must be approved for you. The counseling comes in two phases: initial training and follow-up training.

Your initial training is up to ten hours long; it normally includes one hour of one-on-one counseling followed by up to nine hours of group training, typically in several different sessions. In unusual circumstances, such as deafness or blindness, one-on-ones can replace the group sessions.

The follow-up training must occur in a calendar year after your initial training. Typically it will be a group training session. One-on-one training can be allowed if no group training is available or your doctor or health professional states that you have special needs that must be met. While the session must be at least 30 minutes long, Medicare will pay for up to a two-hour session each year.

Your doctor's office will know about these programs, which are typically given by hospitals and medical centers. The American Diabetes Association can also direct you to programs in your area, just make sure you tell them you want Medicare covered programs.

Topics covered in these sessions are wide-ranging and comprehensive, and include information on nutrition, proper blood sugar testing, managing your blood sugar, dealing with chronic complications caused by diabetes, emotional adjustment to the disease, family support, and community resources.

Nutrition therapy services for diabetics (and some other beneficiaries) discussed in section 2.30 are separate from this service, even though this training service does discuss nutrition.

2.18b Diabetic retinopathy exams

The diabetic retinopathy exams screen the dilated eye to look for retina damage. This is covered every 12 months for those beneficiaries diagnosed with diabetes.

2.19 Dialysis

Medicare covers kidney dialysis.

2.20 Drug abuse and chemical dependency treatment

Drug abuse and chemical dependency treatment is covered under Part B, but it is subject to the mental health limitation discussed in section **1.12**. Covered treatments include psychotherapy, patient education, and possibly limited family counseling.

Note that Part A will cover inpatient stays for treating drug abuse and chemical dependency.

2.21 Drugs and biologicals

Biologicals are agents that come from living organisms, such as vaccines. To avoid confusion, when we discuss drugs in this section, we will include biologicals under that heading as well.

Medicare Part A covers your drugs when you are an inpatient, and Part D covers most of your prescription drugs. Part B does have some coverage of drugs, but it is very specific, and very limited in the case of prescription drugs. Generally, if a drug is covered by Part B, it will not be covered under Part D.

In general, drugs aren't covered under Part B unless they must be administered by a physician or someone under his or her supervision, or it is administered using a covered item of durable medical equipment. This means the drugs are injected or given intravenously. Coverage doesn't depend on the drug itself, but depends rather on how it is administered. Suppose you go to the doctor's office and he or she gives you a shot of penicillin to attack an infection.

He or she might also write you a prescription for penicillin pills to make sure the infection is thoroughly vanquished. In this situation, the shot is covered, but not the prescription — the shot was administered by a doctor, while the pills are self-administered.

Injectable drugs you give yourself, such as insulin, or an injectable drug for a migraine headache, are not covered, again, because they are not given to you by a doctor.

Medicare Part B does pay for some prescription medicines. The few and limited drugs Part B covers are the following, most of which have been established by statute:

- Immunosuppresive drugs and some drugs such as prednisone used with them, but only after a Medicare-covered organ transplant. (If you received a transplant before you became Medicare eligible, it won't pay for the immunosuppresive drugs.)

- Oral anti-cancer drugs. There are just a handful of these; they have both injectable and oral forms. The oral form is covered under Part B:

    ❋ Busulfan (brand name Myleran®)

    ❋ Capecitabine (brand name XELODA®)

    ❋ Cyclophosphamide (brand name Cytoxan®)

    ❋ Etoposide (brand name VePesid®)

    ❋ Melphalan (brand name Alkeran®)

    ❋ Methotrexate

    ❋ Temozolomide (brand name Temodar®)

- Oral antiemetics or antinausea drugs. These drugs are only covered when they help you absorb an anti-cancer medicine, and not just for symptom relief or comfort.

- Erythropoietin (EPO) for some anemic patients on home dialysis who have to inject these drugs. The drugs include Epoetin alfa (Epogen®), and Darbepoetin alfa (Aranesp®).

- Procrit (Epoetin alpha) for some anemic patients who will undergo hip or knee surgery.

- Blood clotting factors for hemophilia patients are covered even when self-administered.

- Intravenous Immune Globulin (IVIG) for home treatment of Primary Immune Deficiency Disease.

- Antigens prepared by a doctor are covered, even in the few cases in which you self-administer these drugs.

As you may recall from the discussion of the home health agency benefit, osteoporosis drugs can be covered by Part B for female beneficiaries who have broken a bone and are under a home health plan of care when these are given by one of the agency's staff to the beneficiary.

A general exception to the rule that Medicare B doesn't cover drugs, is that the durable medical equipment benefit will pay for drugs when it is necessary for you to get the drug through a piece of equipment such as an infusion device or nebulizer. The rules on these are complex and specific because it has to be shown that the equipment is really needed. Having said this, the kinds of drugs that can be administered this way, and thus possibly paid for under Part B, include:

- Anti-cancer drugs

- Narcotics for intractable cancer pain

- Certain antifungal and antiviral drugs

- Inotropic (muscle contraction) drug therapy for chronic heart failure

When you get one of these few Medicare covered drugs from a pharmacy or supplier, and they are enrolled in Medicare, they have to take assignment, and the cost of the drug can never be more than the Medicare approved amount. If you use a non-enrolled pharmacy or supplier, Medicare will pay nothing, and the pharmacy or supplier can charge you anything.

2.22 Eye coverage

Medicare generally does not cover routine eye exams whether they are to check on your eye health or the correctness of your glasses prescription. However, there are exceptions to this:

- Medicare pays for glaucoma screening for those people at high risk for this disease. See section **2.22d** to find out if you qualify; if you do, it's covered every 12 months.

- Medicare pays for diabetic retinopathy exams for those with diabetes; this screening, a dilated eye exam to look for retina damage, is covered every 12 months for those beneficiaries diagnosed with diabetes. See section **2.18b** to find out if you qualify.

2.22a Eye refractions

Eye refractions are tests that ophthalmologists or optometrists give to prescribe glasses or contacts. These tests are not covered, with the exception discussed in section 22.2d.

2.22b Eye treatments

Medicare covers diagnosis and treatment of diseases of the eyes, such as cataracts, macular degeneration, and trauma. These are covered as any other body organ.

2.22c Eyeglasses and contact lenses

Eyeglasses and contact lenses are not covered, with one exception. If you have cataract surgery and you have an implanted lens, Medicare will pay for corrective lenses — either eyeglasses or contact lenses. It will pay for two lenses or contacts even if only one of your eyes was operated on. It will pay only for standard frames if you get glasses. This benefit is available only once for each cataract operation.

If you want to have much nicer frames than the low-budget, standard frames, your ophthalmologist, optometrist, or optician can supply you with your choice of better or deluxe frames if he or she gives and has you sign an Advanced Beneficiary Notice stating that the difference in cost will not be covered by Medicare. You will have to pay for the difference in the cost of the two frames.

2.22d Glaucoma screening

Medicare covers glaucoma screening as a preventative service, but only for those who are at high risk for this disease. Medicare defines high risk as the following:

- You have diabetes.
- You have a family history of glaucoma.
- You are an African-American who is 50 years or older.
- You are a Hispanic-American 65 years or older.

This screening test can be given once every 12 months. The test can be given by physicians and, in many states, optometrists.

2.23 Federally Qualified Health Clinics (FQHCs)

Federally Qualified Health Clinics (FQHCs) are located in medically underserved areas. They offer the services of physicians, physician assistants, nurse practitioners, and several other kinds of health practitioners. They charge a set encounter fee each time you are seen by a health professional, but that fee is the same no matter how many professionals you see during that visit (e.g., if you see a physician and a health nutritionist). You can keep your coinsurance down by seeing all professionals on one visit rather than on several visits. You get a little extra protection this way, because if you have a covered service and a noncovered one, Medicare will still pay the whole fee because at least something was a covered service during your visit, and the fee is due anyway.

Note that lab tests and diagnostic tests are in addition to the encounter fee. The Part B deductible does not apply to any encounter fee charged by one of these clinics.

2.24 Flu vaccine

The influenza (flu) vaccine is a preventative service and Medicare will pay for one vaccine each flu season. This means you can get a shot late in one season, such as in January, and still get another shot that same calendar year in the next season, such as in October. There is no deductible or coinsurance.

Responding to public health concerns, Medicare has bent the rules so that nontraditional providers such as pharmacists and independent nurses can give flu vaccines and bill on a mass basis for them. Be warned that if you get a flu vaccine from a nonparticipating doctor (that is, one that does not always take assignment on Medicare claims), he or she can charge anything he or she wants as vaccines are not subject to the limiting charge.

2.25 Foot care

While Medicare excludes routine foot care as a covered service, it will pay for the services of a physician or a podiatrist for the medically necessary treatment of diseases of and injuries to the foot (e.g., hammer toe, bunion deformities, heel spurs).

Medicare will also pay for more common procedures such as removing corns, calluses, and clipping nails, but only under special circumstances. These circumstances are that the beneficiary has a medical condition such that nonprofessional foot care might be hazardous to his or her health. If a person with a significant circulatory problem in his or her feet has a wound that would not easily heal, or an infection from accidentally cutting himself or herself while removing a callus, he or she could qualify for the exception.

2.26 Hearing aids and hearing exams

Hearing aids are specifically excluded by law from coverage, as is an examination for them or their fitting. However, if a hearing aid is not medically appropriate (e.g., because of a congenital deformity), a cochlear implant or the like may be covered.

Routine screening tests or exams for hearing, or for prescribing or fitting hearing aids, are not covered. Such tests are covered in the unusual case they are needed to properly diagnose an illness or injury.

2.27 Hepatitis B vaccines

Vaccines for hepatitis B are a preventative service. The series of three shots are covered by Medicare for those at medium to high risk for this disease. This includes beneficiaries who —

- have hemophilia;

- have end-stage renal disease;

- are homosexual men;

- are clients of institutions for the mentally handicapped, or those who work there;

- live within the same household as a hepatitis B carrier; or

- are illegal injectable drug users.

Your doctor may also recommend the vaccine if you have a condition that lowers your resistance to infection.

If you need the vaccines because you are traveling abroad, Medicare will not cover them. Vaccines are not covered by the limiting charge rule, so try to use a Medicare participating physician or one who will take assignment.

2.28 Inpatient ancillaries

In the unusual circumstance that you do not have Medicare Part A, or if you have exhausted your Part A inpatient days, the diagnostic tests and therapeutic services you get in a hospital or Skilled Nursing Facility will be covered under Part B as if you got them as an outpatient. For example, if you receive surgery, Part B will help pay for the use of the operating room; if you have a CAT scan, Medicare will cover that. These ancillaries are priced and paid under the hospital outpatient prospective payment system, in which you can end up paying more than 20 percent coinsurance. But, at least you have some significant financial help with your stay.

2.29 Mammograms

Mammograms are covered both as a preventative service and as a diagnostic service. Any female Medicare beneficiary 40 years of age or older can get a mammogram once every 12 months. Note that 11 full months must have passed since the last screening mammogram.

A female beneficiary in the age range of 35 to 39 can get one baseline mammogram. These screening mammograms are not subject to the deductible but you do have to pay the 20 percent coinsurance.

Diagnostic mammograms — those taken because disease is actually suspected — are covered, but the deductible also applies to these as well as coinsurance.

2.30 Nutrition therapy

Medicare will cover nutritional counseling in two limited situations — for diabetics, and for kidney disease patients who are not on dialysis or who have had a kidney transplant. Those people on dialysis are supposed to get appropriate nutritional counseling as part of their dialysis services.

Nutritional counseling can be given by a registered dietitian or by a nutritionist approved by Medicare (be sure to verify that Medicare has approved the person before you get services from him or her). Do not confuse this service with diabetes self-management training, which Medicare will not cover for every diabetic. Every beneficiary diagnosed as a diabetic is eligible for the nutrition therapy service.

Your doctor must prescribe nutrition therapy. Therapy can consist of an initial assessment of your nutrition and lifestyle; counseling on what foods to eat, how to manage lifestyle factors that affect your diet, and follow-up visits to see how well you are progressing in managing your nutrition and diet. Medicare will pay for up to three hours of one-on-one therapy or counseling the first year you use this service, and two hours a year thereafter. Your doctor must prescribe anew for each year you get these services.

You should also be aware that if your diabetic condition changes significantly, Medicare may cover additional counseling sessions to deal with it; of course, your doctor must prescribe these.

2.31 Pap smear, pelvic exam, and breast exam

A pap test (Papanicolaou stain), a pelvic exam, and a clinical breast exam are covered screening services for all women once every 24 months.

For women at high risk for cervical or vaginal cancer, the test and exams are covered every 12 months. High risk in this case is defined as either of two situations:

- The beneficiary is of childbearing age and had an abnormal pap test, or other abnormalities, within the last 36 months.
- Based on medical history or other findings, the beneficiary is at high risk of developing these cancers. For example, the beneficiary —
  * has not had a pap test with the last seven years,
  * has had less than three normal pap tests within the last seven years,
  * is the daughter of a woman who took diethylstilbestrol (DES) during pregnancy,
  * began having sexual intercourse before the age of 16,
  * has had five or more sexual partners in her life, or
  * has had a sexually transmitted disease.

A screening pelvic exam is a complete physical examination of the woman's external and internal reproductive organs, and this is typically done when the pap smear is taken, and the screening breast exam is made at the same time. The frequency rules for all these are the same.

The deductible does not apply to these services, but coinsurance does. The actual pap test itself (as with any lab test) is paid for in full by Medicare.

2.32 Partial hospitalization

Partial hospitalization is an important mental health benefit that can be given by either a hospital outpatient department or a Community Mental Health Center. It is an intense level of treatment designed to either shorten one's psychiatric stay as a hospital inpatient or to prevent a patient's hospitalization because of an episode of mental illness. It generally involves therapeutic care of the patient for extended periods during the day, when the program delivers individual or group therapy, occupational therapy, individual active therapies, and other services, including non-self-administered drugs and family counseling when centered on healing the patient. It is not meant to be anything like an adult day care or a vocational or diversionary program.

Meals, transportation, and self-administered drugs are not covered. Partial hospitalization services are paid at the reduced outpatient mental health rate. (See Section **1.12a**, above)

2.33 Pathology

Pathology is considered the same as lab tests. The lab has to take assignment on all of these tests and Medicare pays 100 percent of the approved charge, without regard to your deductible, so your liability is zero for these services.

2.34 Pneumonia or pneumococcal vaccine

Every year Medicare beneficiaries die from pneumococcal pneumonia, which is almost entirely preventable. All you need is a preventative vaccine and you are protected for life.

Similar to the annual flu vaccine, there is no deductible or coinsurance for the pneumococcal vaccine. Note that in the very unusual instance when it is medically necessary, Medicare will pay for a second vaccine. Again, vaccines are not covered by the limiting charge rule so try to use a Medicare participating physician or one who will take assignment.

2.35 Portable X-rays and diagnostic X-rays

Portable X-ray suppliers can take certain straight-forward X-rays, when these are ordered by a physician, in your residence, or in some types of

provider facilities. Even though these kinds of providers are certified by the Medicare program they can be participating providers, or not, just like doctors. Be sure, if you use one of these, the supplier is participating in Medicare or takes assignment as the limiting charge does not apply.

Diagnostic X-rays are covered.

2.36 Prostate cancer screening

A screening Prostate Specific Antigen (PSA) test and a digital rectal exam are covered every 12 months for all men beginning the day after their 50th birthday. The PSA test itself, as with any lab test, is paid for in full by Medicare, but the usual deductible and coinsurance apply to the collection charge and to the exam.

2.37 Radiation therapy

Radiation therapy is covered. If you get it in a hospital outpatient department, you pay a co-payment. If you get it in a doctor's office or independent clinic, you pay the standard 20 percent coinsurance.

2.38 Rural health clinic (RHC)

Rural health clinics (RHCs) are located in rural, medically underserved areas. They offer the services of physicians, physician assistants, nurse practitioners, and several other kinds of health practitioners. In some instances they can offer nursing visits to a homebound patient.

RHCs charge a set encounter fee each time you are seen by a health professional, but that fee is the same no matter how many professionals you see during that visit (e.g., if you see a physician and a health nutritionist within a few hours of one another, that's one visit, and one encounter fee). Note that lab tests and diagnostic tests are in addition to the encounter fee. The Part B deductible does not apply to any encounter fee charged by one of these clinics.

2.39 Physician second and third opinions

If you decide that you want a second physician's opinion about getting surgery, or even a major diagnostic procedure such as a cardiac catheterization, Medicare will cover its share of this second opinion. If you do consult with another physician, and that physician's opinion differs from the first physician's opinion, then the program will also cover a third physician's opinion.

2.40 Smoking cessation counseling

If you have a disease that is caused or complicated by tobacco use, or if you take a medicine that is affected by tobacco usage, Medicare will cover cessation therapy. Specifically, Medicare will pay for up to eight face-to-face therapy sessions over the course of 12 months.

2.41 Telemedicine

Telemedicine or telehealth in Medicare is where a patient receives services from a health professional located some distance away, and where audio and video equipment is used to permit two-way, real-time interactive communication between the patient and the health professional.

The telemedicine benefit has gradually been expanded in Medicare. The Medicare patient must be in a nonmetropolitan area to qualify. At this time only certain visits are covered, such as office visits, consultations, individual psychotherapy, psychiatric diagnostic interview exams, pharmacological management, some end-stage renal disease related services, and individual medical nutrition therapy, but more will be added to the list over time.

2.42 Transplants

Medicare covers a number of transplant procedures such as the following:

- Bone marrow

- Intestine and viscera
- Lung
- Cornea
- Kidney
- Pancreas (some)
- Heart
- Liver

With the exception of bone marrow and cornea transplants (which are usually given on an outpatient basis), Medicare covers the other transplants named in the list above, but only in specially approved facilities. These are not covered in every Medicare certified hospital, only in ones that are specifically approved for that particular type of transplant. Part A is necessary to cover the hospital costs.

As indicated in section 2.21, one of the few drugs Part B will cover are the immunosuppressive drugs used following a Medicare covered transplant. That is, if Medicare paid for your transplant, it will cover its share of the cost of these expensive drugs.

Also important is that the costs of procuring the organ to be transplanted are covered by a special Medicare program, and there is no cost to you.

2.43 Transportation

Transportation is not covered, other than by ambulance (see section 1.9). Unlike the Medicaid program, which often covers the transportation of patients to medical services when they can't otherwise get there, Medicare has no similar benefit.

Some communities have volunteer transportation programs, so you may wish to seek these out, while some national organizations sponsor local programs. For example, the American

Cancer Society's "Road to Recovery" program assists cancer patients who need help to get to their treatments.

2.44 Vaccinations

While Medicare specifically covers flu vaccines for all beneficiaries, and pneumococcal and hepatitis B shots for those at risk, it does not cover other preventative vaccinations such as for international travel.

Vaccinations covered by Medicare are not subject to the limiting charge rules. Be sure you understand what you will have to pay out-of-pocket for these.

2.45 "Welcome to Medicare" Physical Exam

The only time Medicare covers a routine (non-symptomatic) or wellness examination is the "Welcome to Medicare" exam. You must get this exam within the first 12 months of your entitlement to Medicare Part B, and you get the exam only once.

The exam is specific as to what your doctor will do. Your doctor will record your medical history and check your blood pressure, weight, height; calculate your body mass index (BMI); and screen you for depression. Your doctor should also give you a vision test and an electrocardiogram (ECG) and make sure that you are up-to-date with your vaccinations. Depending on your general health and medical history, your doctor may recommend further tests.

Your doctor will also counsel you to help prevent disease, improve your health, or stay well and give you a written plan (e.g., a checklist) letting you know which screenings and other preventative services you should get. Your doctor will also talk with you about end-of-life planning, including advance directives.

The Part B deductible no longer applies to the "Welcome to Medicare" exam; only the coinsurance applies.

The further tests and additional screening and preventative services your doctor may recommend are not included as part of the "Welcome to Medicare" exam with one exception. If you are referred for an aortic aneurysm ultrasound screening, Medicare will pay its share for that (see section **2.1**). See the Exams for Men and Women tables included on the CD to find out what kinds of tests you can get and when you can get them.

It will probably take some time for you to get an appointment for your exams so don't wait until you have Medicare and then make the appointment. You'll know ahead of time when you'll get Part B, so preschedule your "Welcome to Medicare" exam for when you become a beneficiary. You may as well find out as soon as you are entitled to Medicare how you are doing with your health, what other tests you may need, or even what medical interventions you should have.

Because at the time of this exam you are a new Medicare beneficiary, your record with Medicare is a clean slate so if you had a preventative service that under Medicare you can have only once every 12 months, even if you got it six months before you got your Medicare, it will pay for it. (There are exceptions to this, such as mammograms and the bone mineral density X-ray. Strictly adhere to your doctor's advice on frequency for these screenings.)

Note that the CD has Preventative and Screening Schedulers that list all available Medicare preventative and screening tests.

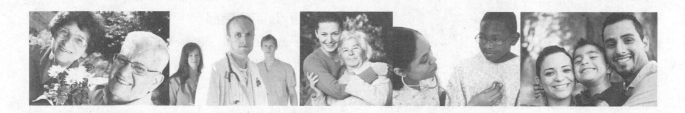

5
Part B: Durable Medical Equipment

The durable medical equipment (DME) benefit is an important part of your Part B benefits, not only because Part B pays for equipment, but you can be covered for most of the items only under specific medical conditions, which are mostly discovered, evaluated, and treated with your general Part B coverage. The equipment must be prescribed or ordered for you by a physician and your visits with the physician are covered under Part B.

This chapter also includes information about prosthetics, orthotics, and supplies. That is because prosthetics, orthotics, and supplies are generally governed by the same rules as medical equipment; claims for these items are processed by the same special claims processors under contract to Medicare to adjudicate durable medical equipment claims, and these items are also subject to special scrutiny as is durable medical equipment.

To qualify as durable medical equipment, an item must be long lasting, used for a medical reason, can't normally be useful to someone who is healthy, and has to be used in your home. Your

doctor has to prescribe the equipment. In the case of durable medical equipment, physician assistants, nurse practitioners, and clinical nurse specialists may also prescribe it.

A durable medical equipment supplier must both be enrolled in Medicare and be a participating supplier for you to be fully protected on what you will be liable for. This is because the limiting charge does not apply to durable medical equipment and supplies. A participating supplier will take assignment on every item of durable medical equipment, and you will be liable for only 20 percent of the Medicare approved charge.

An enrolled supplier who does not participate and who does not specifically take assignment on a particular item can charge you anything it wants, and demand payment up front and in full, even before delivery of the item. This is never good for you. If a supplier is not enrolled with Medicare, Medicare will not pay you or the supplier for any item, even if it is a well-known company. You can always find out if a supplier is participating by going on the Medicare website.

1. Coverage of Durable Medical Equipment

The durable medical equipment benefit covers a variety of equipment and items, prosthetics, orthotics, and supplies. The following sections indicate what may be covered and include some comments for clarification on coverage for particular items or classes of items.

First be aware that many things are *not covered*, which include:

- Air cleaners
- Air conditioners
- Adult diapers
- Bathtub seats
- Dehumidifiers
- Emesis basins
- Face masks
- Home improvements such as ramps or tub rails
- Incontinence pads
- Overbed tables
- Parallel bars
- Reading machines
- Spare oxygen tanks
- Stairway elevators and stair glides
- Surgical stockings or hose
- Telephone alert systems
- Treadmills or other exercise equipment
- Wheelchair lifts for cars
- Wigs
- Whirlpool baths

The following items *are covered.*

Air-fluidized bed

These are used to help eliminate pressure sores and are covered.

Breast prosthesis

This is covered, including a surgical brassiere, after a mastectomy. As this comes from a supplier, be sure the supplier takes assignment.

Canes

Canes are covered, but not canes used by the blind to navigate.

Commode chairs

Commode chairs are covered, but only if you are confined to your bedroom.

Crutches

Crutches are covered.

Diabetes supplies

Part B does not pay for injectable insulin or syringes for diabetes supplies, because even though it is an injectable drug, it is self-administered. However, Part D does cover insulin and syringes.

Medicare does cover the equipment and supplies diabetics need (whether or not they take insulin) to monitor their blood sugar levels. Thus, blood sugar (glucose) monitors, test strips, lancet devices, and lancets are covered. Generally speaking, if you take insulin, Medicare will pay for up to 100 test strips and lancets a month, and a lancet device every six months. If you don't take insulin, Medicare covers up to 100 test strips and lancets every three months, as well as a lancet device every six months. It will pay for glucose control solutions to make sure your testing equipment gives accurate results.

Your physician has to prescribe diabetic supplies (sometimes this is called a dispensing order), and indicate in the prescription that you have diabetes, whether you take insulin, how often you need to test your blood sugar, and how many test strips and lancets you require each month. This prescription also has to specify what kind of a blood monitor you need. In some cases (e.g., low vision or a manual dexterity impairment), Medicare will cover a special monitor to overcome your deficit.

To obtain your diabetic testing supplies, you can either go to or order them from a pharmacy or a durable medical equipment supplier. Because of significant abuse of this particular benefit in the past, there are some unique rules on how you can get these diabetic supplies:

- If you get the supplies from a pharmacy or supplier, you have to order them, your doctor can't.

- You must ask for refills, as your supplier is not permitted to automatically send you supplies. However, they are allowed to remind you to reorder.

- You will have to get a new prescription every year for your test strips.

- The monitor, test strips, and lancets must be billed directly to Medicare by a supplier; this is the one claim you can never send in yourself.

- You must use a participating supplier or pharmacy, or one that will take assignment on your claim, because if it is nonparticipating and it doesn't take assignment, the supplier can charge you anything it wants. You will receive nothing from Medicare if you use a non-enrolled pharmacy or supplier.

Medicare does not cover urine test strips, wipes or swabs, disinfectants (e.g., alcohol or peroxide), or antibacterial skin cleaners.

Dialysis machines

Dialysis machines are covered. If you decide to do home dialysis, you will have to choose whether or not you wish to work with a dialysis facility to get all your services, equipment, and supplies, or whether you want to use a durable medical equipment supplier to do this. These are known in Medicare as "Method I" and "Method II," respectively. You need to know that once you choose a method, you'll have to live with that method for the rest of that calendar year. Suppliers must accept assignment of home dialysis equipment and supplies delivered under Method II.

Drugs

One exception to Part B's noncoverage of drugs and biologicals occurs when the durable medical equipment benefit will pay for drugs when it is necessary for you to get the drug through a piece of equipment such as an infusion device or nebulizer. The rules on these are complex and specific as it has to be shown that the equipment approach is really needed. (This topic is covered more fully in the Chapter 4, section **2.21**.)

When you get one of the Medicare-covered drugs from a pharmacy or supplier, and it is enrolled in Medicare, it has to take assignment, and thus the cost of the drug is never more than the Medicare approved amount. If you use a non-enrolled pharmacy or supplier, Medicare will pay nothing, and the supplier or pharmacy can charge you anything.

External infusion pump

An external infusion pump is a device that is used to administer drugs at a specific rate over a set period of time and, when appropriate, is covered by Medicare, along with the associated drug (e.g., insulin or morphine). See section 4., because submitting a special form will be necessary to get this covered.

Hospital beds

Hospital-type beds for in-home use are covered.

Lymphedema pumps and pneumatic compression devices

Lymphedema pumps and pneumatic compression devices are used to treat either lymphedema or chronic venous insufficiency. Generally, you must have tried progressive therapy before this can be prescribed for you, and it is subject to monthly recertification.

Nebulizers

Nebulizer devices give medicine in the form of a mist to your lungs. The devices and the drugs they use can be covered.

Orthotics

Orthotics are leg, arm, back, and neck braces, including special corsets and belts (e.g., a sacro lumbar corset). The device's design, materials, measurement, and fabrication are covered as well as the fitting, testing, and training. In addition, the cost of adjustment, repairs, and replacements of these devices are also covered. The device is covered by Medicare even if the original device was not paid for by Medicare.

Those who supply these orthotic devices do not have to take assignment and are not subject to the limiting charge, so before you order or are fit for one of these, get a clear understanding of whether the supplier participates or will take assignment, and if not, what you will be liable for.

Osteogenesis stimulators

Osteogenesis stimulators are also called electrical osteogenic stimulators and bone growth stimulators. The stimulators are covered, but see section 4. for information on extra documentation.

Ostomy supplies

Medicare will pay for ostomy supplies, including pouches, irrigation supplies, and holders for those who have had a colostomy, ileostomy, or urinary ostomy and must maintain their stoma. As with any supply, be sure your supplier takes assignment. Normally, Medicare will pay for three months of supplies at a time, unless you are in a nursing home, in which case Medicare will pay one month's supply at a time.

Medicare won't pay for associated ostomy items such as skin lotions, measuring containers, bag holders, pouch covers, and catheter care kits.

Oxygen

One durable medical equipment benefit is supplying oxygen to a beneficiary in his or her home where this is medically warranted. However, because oxygen therapy has been overused and because it can lead to serious adverse events, the medical criteria for this benefit are very clearly defined. The following three criteria must all be met:

- You must be diagnosed with severe lung disease or with certain symptoms that might improve with oxygen therapy (e.g., pulmonary hypertension or nocturnal restlessness).

- You must have tried alternative forms of treatment, which proved to be unsuccessful.

- The specific level of oxygen in your blood must fall below certain levels as determined by a lab test known as a blood gas study.

Your attending physician must document these three situations on a special form (Certificate of Medical Necessity CMS-484 — Oxygen).

Your physician must also specify your oxygen flow rate, how frequently you need to use your oxygen (e.g., ten minutes per hour), and the expected duration of use (e.g., six months or lifetime). This information is kept by your oxygen supplier to document your claim, although in some cases these must be submitted to your Durable Medical Equipment Medicare Administrative Contractor to get your oxygen claims paid or to your Regional Home Health Intermediary if you are getting your equipment and oxygen as a home health benefit.

The specific equipment that you qualify for can include oxygen in gas or liquid form, and the special equipment and vessels needed to safely store and deliver it to you (e.g., tubing).

If you can move about, Medicare will pay for a portable oxygen system to keep you mobile. It won't pay for a portable oxygen system for you to use as a back-up system, or if you require oxygen only during sleep.

Parenteral and enteral nutrition

Parenteral and enteral nutrition are covered under the prosthetic benefit of Medicare Part B, as these types of nutrition therapy are in effect a substitution for a permanently inoperative body organ, meaning the inability of the digestive tract to absorb sufficient nutrients for a beneficiary to maintain weight and strength. Both these nutrition approaches bring an artificial nutrient to the body; the parenteral approach brings it directly into a patient's veins, while the enteral brings it to the alimentary tract through a tube, such as a nasogastric tube.

Coverage for either parenteral or enteral nutrition must be obtained through special documentation submitted by the supplier to the Durable Medical Equipment Medicare Administrative Contractor on a Form CMS-10126 — Enteral and Parenteral Nutrition. If coverage is approved, then the equipment and supplies necessary to infuse the nutrients, as well as the nutrients, are covered under Part B. Typically, the nutrients must be ordered and paid for on a month-to-month basis, while the supplies and equipment are paid for under the usual durable medical equipment rules.

Patient lifts

Patient lifts can be manual or electrical and are typically used to get someone from a bed to a wheelchair and vice versa. The lifts are covered by Medicare.

Power mobility devices

This is a Medicare term for power wheelchairs and power-operated vehicles or scooters. In order to be covered, you have to meet the requirements for getting a manually operated wheelchair (i.e., you have a mobility deficit that cannot be overcome with a cane or walker), but you must also be unable to operate a manual wheelchair, perhaps because you don't have enough upper body strength, endurance, coordination, or range to do so. However, you have to have enough strength and posture control to be able to operate one of these power mobility devices, and do so safely. Your home must be deemed able to accommodate the device as well.

The requirement has to do with mobility related activities of daily living, which include toileting, dressing, feeding, grooming, and bathing. If you have a mobility deficit that restricts you from doing these actions in the customary rooms or areas of your home, puts you at heightened risk when you perform these tasks, or even if they restrict you from completing these activities in a reasonable amount of time, you are considered to have a mobility deficit.

A physician, physician assistant, nurse practitioner, or clinical nurse specialist has to prescribe the power mobility device, and the person must have a face-to-face exam with you to do so. If the person saw you recently as a hospital inpatient, that satisfies this requirement. The exam is covered by Medicare.

There are high costs associated with power mobility devices and Medicare pays for power wheelchairs differently than it does for power-operated vehicles and scooters. It is assumed that you will always get this device from a supplier that takes assignment.

You can choose to purchase a power wheelchair up front. If you elect this, Medicare will pay a lump sum of 80 percent of the approved amount to the supplier, and you will pay 20 percent.

You can elect to rent a power wheelchair. If you do so, Medicare will pay its share (80 percent) and you will pay your share (20 percent) of the rental payments each month for ten months. At that point, you may elect to purchase the power wheelchair. If you do so, Medicare and you will make three more monthly rental payments, and you own it. If you elect not to, Medicare and you will make five more monthly payments, and the supplier will own it.

A beneficiary can choose to rent or purchase a power-operated vehicle or scooter up front. If the beneficiary chooses to rent, Medicare will pay its share of the monthly rental amount up to, but not exceeding, the purchase price. At that point, the supplier, not you, owns the vehicle. If you anticipate needing the vehicle for some time, you should strongly consider the purchase option.

As for maintenance and repair, if you rent, Medicare will pay 80 percent of the allowed amount for service every six months, and you will pay 20 percent. This is true whether or not the item was actually serviced. If purchased, Medicare will pay 80 percent of the approved service charge whenever the vehicle is serviced, and you will pay 20 percent.

Prosthetics

These are devices that replace all or part of a missing, malformed, or inoperative body organ, or one whose function is permanently impaired. Examples include artificial eyes and limbs, a Foley catheter for someone with permanent urinary incontinence, and colostomy bags. The supplies that are needed for the device to work properly, such as batteries for an artificial larynx or flushing supplies for a colostomy, are also covered.

The prosthetic device's design, materials, measurement, and fabrication, as well as the fitting, testing, and training are covered. In addition, the cost of adjustments, repairs, and replacements of a device are also covered. This is true even if the original device was not paid for by Medicare.

Those who supply these devices do not have to take assignment and are not subject to the limiting charge, so before you order or are fit for one of these, get a clear understanding of whether the supplier is participating in Medicare or will take assignment; if not, ask what you will be liable for.

Seat lifts

Seat lifts are mechanisms built into a chair and designed to lower a beneficiary to a sitting position or, vice versa, to raise him or her to a standing position. These can be covered by the Part B durable medical equipment benefit, but only for those who have severe muscular dystrophy or another neuromuscular disease, or severe arthritis of the hip or knee such that, without the device, he or she would be bed or chair confined. All of these situations must be approved by Medicare on a case-by-case basis, using the information in a Certificate of Medical Necessity (specifically, Form CMS-849 — Seat Lift Mechanisms) submitted by your physician to the supplier.

Suction pumps

Medicare covers the cost of suction pumps.

Supplies

Medicare doesn't cover supplies such as first-aid kits, Band-Aids, thermometers, aspirin, or blood pressure meters. However, it does help pay for some medical items of a nondurable kind. These have been covered in the other, more specific entries in this section such as diabetes supplies, ostomy supplies, and home dialysis supplies. The limiting charge does not apply to these supplies, so get supplies from a supplier that participates or will accept assignment on your claim.

Therapeutic shoes or inserts

Medicare will cover therapeutic shoes or special inserts for your shoes under limited circumstances. These circumstances include the following:

- You have severe diabetic foot disease.

- The physician who treats your diabetes certifies that you need the shoes or inserts.

- A qualified doctor or a podiatrist has prescribed the shoes or inserts.

- The shoes or inserts are fitted by a podiatrist, an orthotist, a prosthetist, or a pedorthist.

The Medicare payment covers both the therapeutic shoes or inserts and the fitting of them. In lieu of shoes or inserts, it will pay for modifications that have to be made to your own shoes. These payments are limited to once each calendar year, so if you have these, observe this time frame for when you need changes.

Remember that the limiting charges do not apply to these items, so try to use a participating supplier, or one who will take assignment on your claim.

Traction equipment

Medicare covers traction equipment.

Transcutaneous electrical nerve stimulator (TENS)

Medicare covers transcutaneous electrical nerve stimulators (TENS), which are devices that provide electrical currents through the skin for pain control.

Urological supplies

Urological supplies are covered if you are bladder incontinent or you are unable to eliminate urine when your bladder is full, and either of these conditions is expected to last at least three months. However, Medicare won't pay for associated items such as skin lotions, measuring containers, bag holders, pouch covers, and catheter care kits. Normally Medicare will pay for three months of supplies at a time, unless you are in a nursing home, when it will pay one month's supply at a time.

Ventilators or respiratory assist devices

Medicare will cover ventilators and respiratory assist devices.

Walkers

Medicare will cover walkers.

Wheelchairs

Manually operated wheelchairs are covered if you have a mobility deficit that cannot be overcome with a cane or walker. A mobility deficit has to do with mobility related activities of daily living, which include toileting, dressing, feeding, grooming, and bathing. If you have a mobility deficit that restricts you from doing these activities in the customary rooms or areas of your home, or which puts you at heightened risk when you perform them, or even if the deficit restricts you from completing these activities in a reasonable amount of time, you are considered to have a mobility deficit.

If you need a wheelchair to travel a short distance (e.g., through a shopping mall or a park), it is not covered.

2. Equipment Must Be Supplied to Your Home

One aspect of the durable medical equipment benefit is that the equipment must be supplied to your home.

Any equipment you need while you are in a covered Medicare stay at a Skilled Nursing Facility (SNF) will be covered under your stay by Part A. However, if you are in an SNF in a non-covered stay — perhaps you exhausted your covered days — durable medical equipment is not covered because you are not considered to be in your home. This particular exclusion will also apply to infusion and inhalation drugs delivered by the durable medical equipment supplier and thus normally covered under Part B. However, if you have Part D, that will pay for these drugs.

What's a little confusing is that the "in your home" requirement does not apply to the prosthetics, orthotics, and supplies which are typically associated with the durable medical equipment benefit. Medicare will pay for these items even if you are in an SNF during a non-covered stay. The following are what Medicare will generally pay for in a non-covered stay in an SNF:

- Immunosuppresive drugs
- Refractive lenses
- Orthotics
- Surgical dressings
- Ostomy supplies

- Tracheotomy care kits
- Parenteral and enteral nutrition
- Urological supplies
- Prosthetics
- For end-stage renal disease patients on Method II dialysis, the necessary dialysis supplies

3. Payment Methods for Durable Medical Equipment

It's important for you to know how Medicare pays for durable medical equipment, particularly because with certain items you may be asked to make a decision to rent or to purchase. Basically, Medicare has a fee schedule, which is a list of how much it will approve for each of a whole range of durable medical equipment items and supplies.

Medicare usually pays a monthly rental fee on each item you use. This happens even if you choose the purchase option; its monthly payment is called a monthly rental fee. The fee varies over the time the Medicare program pays it. Specifically, it takes the approved purchase price of the item, and approves 10 percent of that in each of the first three months of use. It then switches to 7.5 percent of the approved purchase price for the rest of the payments. You will see these amounts vary from the beginning to the rest of the payments, and so will your co-insurance amounts, as you will be responsible for 20 percent of each month's approved amount.

Medicare has three general approaches to paying for durable medical equipment, which are discussed in the following sections.

3.1 Low-cost or frequently purchased items

If an item's approved amount is $150 or less, or if the item is one that is normally purchased, then you have the option of purchasing that item up front. The supplier must give you this option. If you take it, when Medicare first gets the claim for this item, it will pay its full share (80 percent of the approved purchase amount) and the supplier will bill you for the other 20 percent. When you take care of your bill, you, and not the supplier, will own the item. (Remember that if you use a supplier that did not take assignment, the supplier can bill you whatever it wants, even above the approved amount.)

You don't have to take the purchase option; if you want, you can go with the rental option. On these items, Medicare will pay only up to and not more than the purchase price. In effect, you will pay the same as if you purchased it up front, but you can make your coinsurance payments monthly.

These low-cost or frequently purchased items include canes, walkers, crutches, commode chairs, blood glucose monitors, pneumatic compressors, and traction devices.

The exception is if you are getting a motorized or power wheelchair, you must be given the option to purchase it up front. If you do purchase it up front, you'll owe the 20 percent coinsurance right away, but you will have no further payments. If you don't, it will be treated as any capped rental item as discussed in section 3.3.

3.2 Always rentals

There are items that Medicare will always make rental payments upon, no matter how long you have the items. These include dialysis units, and items that need frequent servicing, such as ventilators. You will never be given the option to purchase these, and you will have to pay the 20 percent coinsurance on these items every month as long as you use them. On these items, Medicare approves 10 percent of the item's approved purchase price for each of the first three months

of use, and then 7.5 percent of that price for every month that you use the equipment. Medicare pays 80 percent of every approval and you pay 20 percent.

There is an exception for oxygen equipment — Medicare and you will pay a total of 36 payments, and then stop. You, the beneficiary, will then automatically have use of the equipment for another 24 months, which is a total of five years. The supplier will continue to own the equipment, but it is obligated to keep it in good repair and in running order and to furnish any accessories as needed. Medicare will continue to help pay for oxygen that is delivered to this equipment for your use.

After five years of having the oxygen equipment, you will have to decide whether you want to continue with your current supplier. If you do, you begin again with paying rental payments. You will pay 20 percent and Medicare, 80 percent, as usual. Or you can choose a different supplier, and begin the new five-year cycle with it.

Special rules apply if you move away from your supplier's area while it is responsible for your equipment. The supplier has to arrange for you to get equipment and service in your new location at its expense. If you have issues about the transition to this new mandate, or if you move and your supplier doesn't help you, Medicare advises you to call Medicare's toll-free number for assistance. (See the Resources on the CD for the phone number.)

3.3 Capped rental items

For many items, and for most expensive items, Medicare will rent them. Medicare will make a total of 13 payments on the item and then you will own it. Examples of these items include hospital beds and wheelchairs. You, of course, have to pay your normal 20 percent coinsurance on each of these 13 Medicare payments.

Once you own the item, and it needs repair, Medicare will pay its 80 percent share of the approved repair costs, but if the supplier doesn't take assignment on this, your costs will likely be higher.

Caution: If for some reason you decide to buy one of these capped rental items before the 13 months are up, Medicare will not pay anything further for the item.

4. Extra Documentation on Durable Medical Equipment

Special forms need to be submitted for the payment for certain items of durable medical equipment. Specifically, the following list includes the currently required Certificates of Medical Necessity (CMN) that your physician must send to your supplier before you can get Medicare to help pay for these items:

- Form CMS-484 — Oxygen (This is for any home oxygen equipment or gasses.)

- Form CMS-846 — Pneumatic Compression Devices (This is for treating lymphedema or chronic venous insufficiency.)

- Form CMS-847 — Osteogenesis Stimulators (This device promotes bone growth.)

- Form CMS-848 — Transcutaneous Electrical Nerve Stimulator (TENS) (This is needed only if you want to purchase the stimulator.)

- Form CMS-849 — Seat Lift Mechanisms

The following are currently required durable medical equipment information forms (DIF) that your supplier has to send to its special carrier:

- Form CMS-10125 — External Infusion Pumps

- Form CMS-10126 — Enteral and Parenteral Nutrition

5. Advanced Determination of Medical Coverage

You, as a beneficiary, have the right to ask for a decision from Medicare as to whether or not it will pay for certain items of durable medical equipment before you agree to purchase or rent them. Your supplier also has the right to ask for the determination of coverage, and the inquiry is typically made by the supplier rather than the beneficiary.

These determinations are made by the special outfits that process durable medical equipment claims, the Durable Medical Equipment Medicare Administrative Contractors. These decisions can be made only on a limited range of items, specifically, only on those items which are customized for you, and which are expensive. This is good protection for you because if you begin renting a standard item of durable medical equipment and Medicare doesn't cover it, you can tell the supplier to take it back and you are out only a month's rental. However, with customized items, this would be an issue.

To get one of these decisions, you need to make a written request. While no specific form or format is prescribed for these requests, you must include adequate written information from your medical record to identify the customized item and describe what its specific intended use is for you. Your letter must also contain details on your medical condition and why you require the use of the customized item. It might be helpful to include a signed statement that the Medicare Administrative Contractor can contact your physician directly with any questions.

Once this information is submitted, the Medicare Administrative Contractor has 30 calendar days to make a decision; and the contractor has to notify you of the decision in writing. If the Medicare Administrative Contractor decides in your favor and says the item will be covered, this decision is good for six months. If the contractor decides it will not be covered, you have no appeal rights, as this determination is not technically a formal claims decision. At this point you have to decide if you can do without the item, or go with a substitute covered item. If you decide to go ahead and order the item, you will be liable for the payments on the item, but you can have your durable medical equipment supplier submit a formal claim. This claim will almost certainly be denied, but you can then appeal through all the formal appeals steps. (See Chapter 14 for more information on appeals.)

6. If You Leave Original Medicare and Go to Medicare Advantage

If you are in Original Medicare and you join a Medicare Advantage managed care or health plan, you need to contact your plan and ask it to take over the payments, as Original Medicare will stop its monthly payments as of the effective date of your membership in your plan (this is always the first of the month). Also, if you change plans, contact your new plan to make these arrangements.

My experience is that plans tend to control this benefit much more tightly than Original Medicare, and the plan provider may not always want to cover your equipment. Or it may use a supplier that is not your current one, and may make you change to get a better deal.

Conversely, if you are in a Medicare Advantage managed care or health plan and leave it to go to Original Medicare, you need to tell the company that supplied you with whatever durable medical equipment you are renting or purchasing to begin billing Original Medicare as of the date you leave your Medicare Advantage Plan.

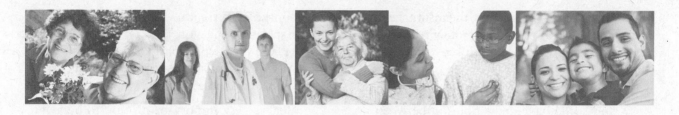

6
Part D: The Prescription Drug Benefit

The Prescription Drug Benefit, or Part D of Medicare, is the newest part of the program. In order to be eligible for Part D, you have to have either Part A or Part B (or both). Just like with Part B, you'll pay a monthly premium; the national average monthly premium was $28 in 2009.

You should understand that you can get Part D coverage either as a stand-alone drug plan, or through a Medicare Advantage or managed care plan (discussed in more detail in Chapter 8). If you can't get Part D as part of your Medicare Advantage or managed care plan, you can sign up with a stand-alone Part D plan and get the prescription drug benefit.

This chapter discusses the Part D benefit from the point of view of stand-alone drug plans. You should understand that Part D drug plans that are part of your Medicare Advantage or managed care plan work the same way as the stand-alone drug plans. You should also be aware that while every stand-alone drug plan requires you to pay a premium (unless you have certain levels of extra help, discussed in Chapter 7), this is not true with all Medicare Advantage Plans.

1. The Part D Structure

Part D was structured to pay for just about all types of prescription drugs and biologicals. Note that the dollar amounts change each calendar year; the following amounts are for 2010:

- **Deductible:** The beneficiary pays for the first $310 in drugs.

- **Basic benefit:** Part D pays for 75 percent and the beneficiary pays for 25 percent of the next $2,520 in drugs.

- **Coverage gap:** The beneficiary pays 100 percent of the next $3,610 for drugs.

- **Catastrophic:** Part D pays for 95 percent and the beneficiary pays for 5 percent of all the rest, with no limit until the end of the calendar year.

The law allows any insurance company or drug plan that wants to offer this benefit the option of sticking to that structure, or of offering one that is the actuarial equivalent, or of structuring their own Part D plan so that the beneficiaries and the government would pay the equivalent dollar amounts. In many cases, the insurance plans that are offered to you only remotely resemble the government's proposed structure; for example:

- Some drug plans have no deductible, but many do have the full $310 deductible, and some have deductibles in between no deductible and the $310.

- Some plans make you pay a straight dollar co-payment for certain drugs and not a percentage or coinsurance amount.

- Some plans will help pay for your drugs through the coverage gap; that is, you can get at least some coverage. No state has fewer than 9 such stand-alone plans as of 2010.

The monthly premiums for stand-alone plans have a range in 2010 from a low of $8.80 in Oregon and Washington, to a high of $120.20 in Delaware, the Distirct of Columbia, and Maryland. To find out this information for your state, see the Medicare Stand-Alone Drug Plans sheet, included on the CD. Note that costs listed in the chart were accurate as of 2010. Medicare sets the Part D premium so that you pay 25 percent of the costs of the Part D prescription drug insurance program. In 2010, the average monthly premium is about $32 per month, but the amounts can vary widely depending on the drug plan you choose.

The general requirement in Medicare Part D is that a drug plan does not have to have all possible drugs in its formulary (formulary means a list of the specific drugs that a drug plan will help pay for). Rather, the rule is that for every type or category of drug that is used to treat a particular medical condition, the plan has to have at least two different drugs. For example, one therapeutic class of drugs could be antifungals; the formulary would have to include at least two different drugs, such as Fluconazole and Ketoconazole, to treat it. With a few exceptions, if the specific drug you take is not on the formulary, the plan won't pay for it. Note also that all Part D plans must have complete and current formularies available on their websites.

What is very important for you to be aware of is that drug plans are allowed to change their formularies. It is possible that when you signed up for your plan that it had one of your medications listed on its formulary, but it was later removed from the list. If you are using the drug, the drug plan has to tell you it is removing the drug from its formulary at least 60 days in advance. If the plan does not give you this notice, your drug plan has to tell you and provide a 60-day supply of the drug. Also note that the price the plan charges for any drug may change at any time.

1.1 Deductible

Part D is structured so that it is expected that each beneficiary has an annual deductible of $310 (in 2010). This deductible will likely go up each year. While many drug plans have the $310 deductible, many plans have arranged their benefits so that you do not have to meet any deductible, or they have set their deductible at a lower amount (e.g., $100). The plans with no deductible tend to have higher monthly premiums.

Note that some plans may have a deductible only for brand name drugs; you may not need to pay it for generic drugs.

1.2 Basic benefit

The basic benefit is where the Part D plan requires you to pay 25 percent of the next $2,520 (in 2010) for drug costs, while your plan pays 75 percent. After your deductible you will find that your plan will pick up a large share of your prescription drug costs.

1.3 Coverage gap

If you have gone past the basic benefit stage, you have then reached the coverage gap stage, which many people call the "donut hole." The coverage gap stage means you are responsible for 100 percent of the drug costs of the next $3,610 (in 2010). That is, you are on your own and the benefit coverage returns only after you reach a total in drug costs of $6,440, of which you would pay $4,550 out-of-pocket. Your out-of-pocket share is the $310 deductible, 25 percent of the basic benefit (i.e., $630), and all of the coverage gap of $3,610, for a total of $4,550.

Some drug plans do provide coverage through this gap, but that coverage is generally restricted to generic drugs. The plans that provide coverage tend to have expensive co-payments or high coinsurance percentages for what they do cover. Some people need this coverage, especially if they're paying more than $350 a month for drugs.

You should keep in mind that often the coverage gap offered by Medicare Advantage or managed care plans is better than what you might be able to get from a stand-alone drug plan.

1.4 Catastrophic coverage

One of the really excellent aspects of Part D is its catastrophic protection. Again, the intended formal structure calls for the plan to pay 95 percent of costs, and you pay 5 percent, once your out-of-pocket expenses reach $4,550 (and total drug costs of $6,440). This is good news for those people on very expensive prescription medications.

Just so you know, the formal structure for this stage calls for you to pay a minimum of $2.50 for a generic or similar drug and $6.30 for others, so you may pay more than 5 percent while in this catastrophic stage, depending on your drug plan's particular benefit structure.

1.5 Tiered payments

One feature that almost all Part D drug plans have is what is called tiered payments. The basic concept here is that instead of a single co-payment amount or coinsurance percentage for all drugs, less expensive drugs have lower co-payments or coinsurance percentages, and the more expensive drugs have higher co-payments and coinsurance percentages. The dividing line is not only what the drug costs, but also what type of drug it is. This is done to encourage you to use less expensive drugs because your out-of-pocket costs will be less (and so will Medicare's).

You will most often see a four-tier system, although some plans have up to six tiers:

- First tier is usually generic drugs, which have the lowest co-payment amount.

- Second tier is preferred name-brand drugs, meaning a brand name drug of a certain therapeutic class that the plan has possibly gotten a good deal on from its manufacturer.

- Third tier includes the non-preferred, name-brand drugs.

- Fourth tier is composed of specialty or high-cost drugs.

It's typical for the co-payments or coinsurance amounts to differ depending at what spending stage you are in (i.e., deductible, basic benefit, coverage gap, or catastrophic). This makes sense because the overall structure of the benefit calls for differing payment levels at differing stages. Plans often mix and match co-payment dollar amounts with coinsurance percentages in the different payment stages, and even at times in the same one.

1.6 Calculating your true out-of-pocket costs

If you fill a prescription and the price of the drug is $25 and you still have to meet your deductible for the calendar year, you will pay the pharmacy $25 for the drug, which is your "true out-of-pocket" cost. This is so even if the retail price your pharmacy charges other customers is $45, the price your drug plan establishes for the drug is the basis for what counts toward your true out-of-pocket cost.

For example, suppose you have satisfied your drug plan's deductible, and you go to get the same drug the next month, and you have to pay 25 percent coinsurance. Your true out-of-pocket cost will be $6.25 (25 percent of $25). The $6.25 is what will count toward your true out-of-pocket cost.

A drug has to be on your plan's formulary for it to count toward your true out-of-pocket costs. If it's not on the formulary, it does not count. You have to pay for it all by yourself and it will not count toward meeting your deductible. For instance, if you pay $50 for a drug and it is not on your plan's formulary, your true out-of-pocket cost is zero; even though you paid $50, nothing is counted toward your deductible!

If other insurance pays for part or all of a cost of a drug, its payments do not count toward your true out-of-pocket cost. For example, suppose you are in the coverage gap stage of your Part D plan, and your plan is one that pays for nothing in this stage. You also have another insurance that pays a flat fee of $20 toward a prescription. If you buy a $25 drug, your insurance will pay $20, and you will pay only $5. It is only this $5 that will count toward your true out-of-pocket costs. At this rate it will take you forever to get out of the $3,610 (in 2010) coverage gap. However, this is not all bad if you are only paying $5 per prescription.

There are some exceptions, and some payments made by others will count toward your true out-of-pocket costs. These include those payments made by the following:

- A family member, friend, or charitable organization (e.g., if your daughter picks up your prescription and pays your co-insurance, this is counted)

- Your health savings account, medical savings account, or flexible spending account

- By a State Pharmacy Assistance Program (only a limited number of states have these)

- Co-payments you may have to make to a Pharmaceutical Manufacturer's Patient Assistance Program (you should call your Part D plan and ask how to report these to it)

- If a pharmacy waives or lowers the amount due for a drug, you are supposed to pay on an individual basis; what the pharmacy pays will generally be what you will pay

- If a pharmacy is offering a general discount on a particular drug and you would pay less using its discount than you would have buying it though your Part D plan, or if you can use a discount card to get a drug for less than you would get it through your plan, what you do pay in these situations will count toward your true out-of-pocket costs (call your plan and ask how to report this)

2. Enrollment Periods and Penalties

Just like the optional Part B, if you don't sign up for Part D when you first can enroll, which was either January 1, 2006 or when you first become entitled to Medicare after that date, you then have to wait for an enrollment period to get it and you will pay a penalty on your premium. The penalty is about 32 cents a month for each month you could have been signed up but were not. Unlike Part B, Medicare will not automatically enroll you in Part D — you have to enroll yourself in a particular drug plan if you want Part D coverage.

If you have prescription drug coverage from some other insurance plan, employer coverage, or union coverage, Medicare law says that the other insurance provider for prescription drugs has to let you know whether or not what you have is *creditable coverage*, that is, whether the coverage you now have is at least as good as Medicare Part D. If you have creditable coverage from your insurance provider, you can continue with it, and you probably won't need to get Part D.

If you have creditable coverage, but you lose it (e.g., your former employer goes bankrupt), you will have an opportunity to sign up for Part D when you lose your other coverage and you will not pay a penalty on your premium. Chances are that your creditable coverage will continue. This is because the law that authorizes the Part D benefit also mandates that the Medicare program will subsidize your employer or union so that it continues to cover your prescriptions.

If your coverage is not creditable, you will probably want to get Part D. This is because if you don't get it when you can, you will have limited opportunities to sign up for it later, and you will be subject to the penalty.

You also need to understand that if you don't have any drug plan, when you go to the drugstore you will pay a high price for your drugs. In other words, the price you get when you are in a plan is one that the plan has negotiated with its presumably hefty buying power to be the best it can obtain. You don't have any such power when you are out on your own, and you can be charged anything. My advice is that even if your prescription drug costs are currently low, if at all possible, you should buy the lowest cost drug plan you can. That way you will never have to pay a penalty on your premium. Illness often sets

in suddenly, and the prescription drugs to cure it or help you can be very expensive. Every calendar year you can change your plan to get the best deal for your particular circumstances.

If you do have drug costs that are higher than about $250 a year, the way the plans are structured you can almost certainly find a plan that will reduce your drug costs. The issue is to figure out which one of the many plans is best for you. The Medicare website includes a section on prescription drug coverage with a tool that can help you find the best plan in your state that will work for you, or you can call Medicare.

You can't get Part D whenever you decide you want it. The enrollment periods are discussed in the following sections. For every enrollment period, you should be aware of when you can sign up and exactly when your enrollment becomes effective.

2.1 Individual initial enrollment period

You always get an individual initial enrollment period, which is basically when you first become entitled to either Part A or Part B. This period is similar to the Part B individual initial enrollment period — you may sign up for Part D in the three months before, the month of, and the three months after you first become entitled to Medicare. If you sign up in the three months before, you will get Part D the month you become entitled to Medicare. If you sign up the month you get your Medicare, or any of the next three months, you will get it the first day of the month after you sign up.

If you retroactively become entitled to Part A or enrolled in Part B, you have a Part D initial enrollment period based on the month in which you received notice of your retroactive entitlement or enrollment and including the following three months. For example, suppose you are notified on March 17, 2010, that your entitlement to Part A and Part B is effective on February 1, 2010. Your initial enrollment period for Part D is March 1 to June 30 of 2010. You will begin with Part D the first day of the month after you sign up with a drug plan during your initial enrollment period.

If you sign up anytime during your initial enrollment period, you will not get charged with a premium penalty.

2.2 Annual coordinated enrollment period

The annual coordinated enrollment period is the period from November 15 to December 31 of every year. During this period, anyone with Part A or Part B can enroll in Part D by signing up with a drug plan, change from one drug plan to another, or withdraw from a drug plan. Every year you need to take this opportunity to make sure you are getting the best Part D drug coverage you can.

Avoid last-minute decisions. If you wait until late December to join or switch plans, you may have more difficulty getting your drug plan's identification card on time and having your premium withheld. You can enroll in a plan or switch plans beginning November 15, with an effective date of January 1. This is also the time you can join a Medicare Advantage health plan or managed care plan (Part C), or switch health plans. Many of these also have drug coverage.

Every October you will receive an Annual Notice of Change from your Part D plan. This document highlights the significant changes that the plan will be making effective on January 1 of the next year. These changes can include additions or subtractions to the plan's formulary; raising or lowering its premiums; and changing its benefit structure, including deductibles, co-payments, tier arrangements, and utilization controls.

You need to go through the notice carefully to figure out if you want to stay with your plan or change to another plan. You can't do this without knowing what other plans offer. Instead of an Annual Notice of Change, it is also possible for you to get a termination letter from your plan, saying that it will discontinue its plan beginning January 1. If this happens, you need to start looking for a plan that will be good for you and join it before January 1.

In mid-October of every year the Centers for Medicare & Medicaid Services will make available appropriate data about each Part D drug plan that will be available in your state beginning the next calendar year. It does its best to get this information posted on its website as soon as possible.

Even though you will likely be besieged by marketing material from your current drug plan and its competitors, you need to do two things:

- Research what other plans are available to you and what they will be offering. You can do this by downloading (from the Medicare website) the comparison of drug plans.

- Wait to get a copy of your red, white, and blue *Medicare & You* handbook, which is updated each year and mailed to each Medicare household. This booklet is tailored to your specific area.

You need to decide what the best plan is for you. Do this by making sure that the list of prescriptions you usually take is completely up-to-date, and then go on the Medicare website's drug plan comparison tool, fill in all your current prescription information, and see what plans are best for you. You can also call Medicare for this information. It may turn out that the plan you currently have continues to be the best for you. If you have had a good experience with your current plan, you should stay with it.

Knowing the exact medicines you take (as well as the dose of each), how often you take the medicines, and your monthly cost can help you decide which Medicare prescription drug plan might be best for you. It is always wise to have a complete, up-to-date list of all your prescriptions available in one place to discuss them with your doctor or pharmacist, or to have, if needed, in an emergency situation. On the CD you will find a Prescription List form to help you catalog your prescription information.

If you see a plan that does a better job at covering the specific drugs you take, don't hesitate to change drug plans. It is easy to change plans by going to the Medicare website or calling Medicare to enroll in a new plan. If you switch to a new drug plan, you will automatically be disenrolled from your current plan on January 1; you don't have to contact your old plan. You should get your new drug plan card in the mail with your brochure, and beginning on January 1, you will be switched to your new plan.

You will have to make sure your pharmacy has the new information about your plan. If you had a mail-order arrangement with your old plan, you will need to set up this arrangement with your new plan. To do this you may have to ask your physician to write new prescriptions for three-month supplies, but your physician has to do this periodically anyway, and it's a good opportunity to renew and update your prescriptions.

2.3 Special enrollment periods

There are special enrollment periods that allow you to sign up for Part D outside the usual enrollment periods when something happens to you. In many cases, you will be notified if you are provided with a special enrollment period,

and informed how to take advantage of it. If you find yourself in a situation in which you had Part D but you somehow lost it, and you can't get it now, ask Medicare for a special opportunity to enroll.

You can get a special enrollment period if you lose coverage from the following:

- Medicaid
- State Pharmacy Assistance Program
- Program of All-Inclusive Care for the Elderly (PACE)

The following sections discuss some of the more common situations in which you will get a special enrollment period.

2.3a Moving outside your drug plan's area

If you permanently move out of your drug plan's service area, you must join one of the drug plans in your new area if you want to stay in Part D. Even if you move between states, your plan may still exist in your new state. For example, if you move from New Hampshire to Maine, you won't need to (and won't have then opportunity to) change your plan, but if you move from New Hampshire to Vermont, you have to change your plan. Medicare combined some states together so that the drug plans would be made available to a substantial beneficiary population. Your drug plan's brochure will tell you what its service area is, or you can call and ask.

Your special enrollment period depends on when you move and when you notify your drug plan of your move. If you notify your drug plan in advance of your move, your enrollment period begins the month before your move and lasts two months from the month when you give notice or when you actually move, whichever is later. If you notify your drug plan after you move, your enrollment period begins with that month and continues for two more months.

"Notify" means when your drug plan actually receives the information about your move, which can be different from the month you mail it. You can call your drug plan, which makes your notification date the actual day of your call.

You must tell your old plan of your move as you must be disenrolled from it six months after you move out of its service area. This will happen automatically if you decide to join a new Part D plan or a Medicare Advantage or managed care plan with Part D coverage. If you choose not to join a new plan, you will lose your Part D coverage.

The effective date of your enrollment can't be before the month of your move (unless you happen to move on the first of a month, as some people do) and it can't be before the month the drug plan gets your notice of relocation. Within these constraints, it will be the three months following the month the drug plan gets your notice, and it should tell you what dates you can elect to actually make the change. You can send your notice of relocation to your old drug plan, or even to the one you now wish to join.

For example, suppose you move on March 15, and you notify your drug plan ahead of time on February 10. Your special enrollment period begins February 1 and lasts until two months after you move, or May 31. You can elect to change plans on April 1, May 1, or June 1.

Another example: Suppose you move on March 15, but you notify your drug plan after the move, on May 10. Your special enrollment period begins on May 1 and goes through July 31. You may elect to change your plan on June 1, July 1, or August 1.

This special enrollment period also applies even if you don't have Part D and make a move to a place where different Part D plans are available from where you used to live.

2.3b Loss of creditable coverage

If you involuntarily lose your creditable health-care coverage (e.g., employment coverage from your current employer or union), you get a special enrollment period to sign up for a Part D plan. Note that if you lose your coverage because you decide to drop it or you didn't pay your health plan premiums, this is considered voluntary disenrollment, not involuntary, and you do not receive a special enrollment period.

Your special enrollment period begins the month you are notified that your coverage ends (or it is reduced to the extent that it is no longer creditable) and continues for the next three months. (Note that your former plan is required to notify you of the termination or reduction.) In that four-month period you may sign up for a Part D plan, and your coverage will begin on the first of the month after you sign up.

You should definitely sign up right away because there is a quirky rule that in order not to get a penalty, you have to become enrolled within 63 days; this will usually fall within your special enrollment period, but not always. Sign up for an effective date for Part D no longer than two months after you lose your creditable coverage.

Also, if you received bad information as to whether or not you had creditable coverage, you can ask for a special enrollment period, and you may also ask that any premium penalty caused by this be waived.

2.3c Employer group health plan changes

Both employers and unions can sponsor employer group health plans. You can be covered by these health plans if you are working or retired from work. These plans may disenroll you (e.g., maybe you lost your job with the company) or give you the opportunity to enroll (e.g., you start working for a company that has a plan). Usually these plans allow you to make changes only at certain times.

If you join up with or resign from an employer group health plan, Medicare gives you the opportunity to deal with Part D. For instance, if you are in Part D, but then sign up with another plan, you can drop your Part D. Or if you leave a plan and you don't have Part D, you can sign up for Part D.

To dovetail the Part D change with your employer group health plan, Medicare allows you to make the Part D change in the same time frame that your employer or union gives you to change its plan. For flexibility, Medicare gives you the choice of any of the three months after your plan's change to make your Part D change effective.

You might decide to resign from your employer's plan because its premiums became too high. For example, suppose your employer group health plan announces its new benefit and rate structure on September 1 and gives everyone until September 30 to decide to make changes with the changes effective October 1 (which is the beginning of the company's new fiscal year). You decide to change to a plan that does not include drug coverage, and also sign up for Part D. You must sign up for Part D by September 30, but you can choose to begin your Part D drug coverage on October 1, November 1, or December 1.

Of course, you should always be exceptionally cautious in choosing to resign from your employer's plan. It is extremely important for you to know that some plans will disenroll you if you sign up for Part D. Even worse, they may also disenroll your spouse, and they may even prohibit you from ever rejoining their plan. Before you enroll in Part D, check carefully with your employer, union human resources people, or the health plan administrator to see what will happen if you enroll in Part D.

2.3d Admitted or discharged from a nursing home or long-term care facility

Note that the term "long-term care facility" includes nursing homes, Skilled Nursing Facilities, rehabilitation, psychiatric, long-term care hospitals (and hospital units), and intermediate care facilities.

There is a special enrollment period on admission or discharge from one of these facilities. The special enrollment period gives you the opportunity to sign up for a drug plan and to disenroll from one. For example, if a beneficiary goes into a psychiatric hospital for a long but indeterminate stay to treat acute depression, the beneficiary will get all of his or her medicines from the hospital, not from his or her drug plan, so the beneficiary may wish to disenroll while he or she is an inpatient and not pay the monthly Part D premiums. When he or she is discharged, the beneficiary can go back to a drug plan under Part D, either the one he or she used before, or another one. Note that the premium penalty will apply in this situation. (Premium penalties are discussed in more detail in section 2.4.)

2.3e Trial periods with Medicare Advantage Plans

Medicare wants to increase enrollment in its Medicare Advantage managed care and health plans (Part C), and to do this it has somewhat dovetailed the enrollment process for managed care with Part D. As the open enrollment seasons for both are the same (i.e., November 15 through December 31 every year), you can elect to go into a Medicare Advantage managed care or health plan and get Part D with that plan at the same time, even if you don't have Part D at the time you sign up with the plan.

To encourage you to at least try managed care, Medicare has set up two Part D special enrollment periods to make sure that, if you go into managed care to try it out and you decide you don't like it, you can go back to Original Medicare and join a stand-alone drug plan (i.e., a plan not part of the managed care organization). Even more importantly is that with both of these trials you may also have the guaranteed right to get a Medigap policy, which you will probably need if you are in Original Medicare and have no other insurance. The two trial periods include the following:

- You drop your Medigap policy to try managed care and then leave the plan. If you dropped your Medigap policy when you went into Medicare Advantage or managed care plan, you can get it back and get Part D too. Specifically, if you drop a Medigap policy when you enrolled in a Medicare Advantage Plan for the very first time, and you leave your managed care plan within 12 months of joining it, you may enroll in a Part D stand-alone drug plan and you have the right to a guaranteed issue to buy a Medigap policy. This rule applies no matter how long you were a Medicare beneficiary before you went into managed care.

- Special enrollment period at age 65. This provision affects you if you enroll in Medicare managed care in your seven-month initial enrollment period for managed care: the month you turn 65, and three months on either side of that month. In other words, if you turn 65 in April, your seven-month initial enrollment period runs from January to July. The general rule is that when you first turn 65 and have Medicare, you have an initial enrollment period to join a Medicare managed care plan. If you do enroll in

managed care at this point and then leave it within 12 months after you are in it to go into Original Medicare, you can also join a Part D stand-alone drug plan. In this case you also get a period in which you have the right to a guaranteed issue of a Medigap policy whether or not you previously had one. You must sign up for it with the Medigap insurer in the time frame, beginning with the 60 days before your enrollment in a Medicare Advantage or managed care plan ends, and ending 63 days after you leave. So, for example, if you leave your Medicare Advantage plan on October 1, you have from August 2 until December 2 (60 days before and 60 days after) to obtain a Medigap policy.

To a certain extent these Medigap protections are more important than the protection for Part D; you can sign up for Part D at least once a year, but that is not true with guaranteed issue of Medigap policies in most states.

2.3f Erroneous or misleading information

If you can show that you received erroneous information that caused you not to sign up for a plan (maybe you were wrongly told you had creditable coverage), you may be able to get a special enrollment period to cover this problem. You will need to contact Medicare and request this.

2.4 Penalties

If you do not enroll in Part D at your first opportunity (i.e., during your initial enrollment period), or if you drop it and sign up for it again later, you will probably have to pay a premium penalty. This is assuming you did not have creditable coverage. Specifically, the penalty is 1 percent for each month you could have been enrolled but were not. For example, you could have enrolled on July 1, 2007, but you did not sign up until December 7, 2009, with an effective date of January 1, 2010. You will be assessed a penalty of 30 percent, or 1 percent a month for each of the 30 months you could have had Part D but did not. There is no limit on how high this percentage can go.

The actual penalty is based not on the premium that you must pay your Part D plan, but on a national average monthly premium, which the actuaries at the Centers for Medicare & Medicaid Services calculate for each calendar year — for 2010, it was $31.94. Your penalty is: $31.94 x 30 percent = $9.60 per month (rounded to the nearest 10 cents).

The penalty is refigured every year when the new Part D premiums go into effect. This is calculated by multiplying the new national average premium amount by your applicable penalty months. Seeing that the premiums typically go up, the penalties get worse every year even though your penalty percentage remains the same.

This emphasizes the need to sign up as soon as you can to avoid these significant penalty increases. Unlike the Part A premium penalty, the penalty never expires for Part D.

If you qualify for extra help (also called the low-income subsidy) and have to pay part of your premium, you do not have to pay any penalty on your premium. This is true even if you had a penalty and then became qualified for this. (See Chapter 7 for more details on extra help.)

2.5 Premium payments

When you choose a Part D plan, you also choose how to pay your premium. You can have it deducted from your monthly Social Security, Railroad, or Federal retirement payment. Or you can choose to pay your drug plan directly every month, and some plans allow automatic withdrawal from your checking account. One problem is that if you sign up late in an enrollment period (e.g., December 26), it's too late to take your January premium out of your January Social Security payment. This means you'll get deducted two months' premium in February.

Note that if you have asked for your premiums to be withheld, your plan can't direct-bill you to catch up if there has been a delay. If your plan has been directly billing you, it can't terminate you for nonpayment of premiums until it has notified you of your obligation. If you are in arrears other than you have just refused to pay your premium, your plan has to give you as many months as there is an arrearage to catch up (e.g., if you are four months in arrears, you get four months to catch up.)

3. Pharmacy Networks

One area of concern you may have is whether your pharmacy works with Part D. In general, large pharmacies and stores such as Walgreens, Rite Aid, and Wal-Mart will take any Part D drug plan. However, many smaller independent pharmacies will deal with only a select few plans. The Medicare web program will let you name a particular pharmacy so you can see if it works with whatever plan looks good to you. This info is usually also on the plan's website, or you could check with your pharmacist. Note that specifying a particular pharmacy when choosing a drug plan may reduce the number of plans available to you and that you may not get the best deal you otherwise could with more choices of pharmacies. Having flexibility with your choice of pharmacy will reduce your drug costs, sometimes considerably.

You should be cautioned that some stores and pharmacies have connections to certain companies offering drug plans, so the advice you get from them won't necessarily be best for you in picking a plan. Again, use the Medicare.gov tool to find the best plan for you.

Be aware that if you have to buy a drug from a pharmacy that is not part of your drug plan's network (e.g., when traveling out of state), you will probably have to pay the difference between what you would have paid in-network and what you are charged by the out-of-network pharmacy, along with any co-payment or coinsurance your plan normally makes you pay. If you use the national pharmacies and big chain stores, you'll probably stay in-network and avoid the extra costs.

4. Mail Order

One feature that many beneficiaries find incredibly convenient is that most Part D plans have a mail-order service. If your physician writes you a prescription, you can buy the drugs you use routinely in three-month supplies, and all through the mail.

Some plans, if you use their mail service, will waive one of the three months' co-payments. By using mail order, you have fewer trips to the drugstore and you can usually renew by calling a toll-free number, and the mail order people use your credit card number to charge your co-payment. Not only is it convenient, it might be less expensive than filling your prescriptions once every month. One caution: Be sure to call in plenty of time for them to ship your order.

If your plan doesn't offer a mail-order feature, you may want to find a plan that does.

5. Utilization Controls

You should be aware that Part D drug plans are permitted to employ a whole range of techniques to limit the particular type and quantity of drugs they authorize you to have under their particular plan. It's possible that you will never come across these techniques, but in case you do, here are a few examples:

- **Generic substitution:** Providing the generic equivalent of a drug instead of the prescribed drug (usually brand name).

- **Number of pills:** It may limit the number of pills or doses of a medicine it will permit you to have in a given time period — usually in a month.

- **Prior authorization:** It may require your prescribing physician to call the drug plan and get approval for a specific medicine.

- **Step therapy:** This is sometimes also known as the Fail First Requirement. You may be required to try a certain, usually less expensive, drug to see if it is effective for your condition, and your plan will pay for an alternate drug only if the first one does not work for you.

6. Medication Therapy Management Programs

One thing you should be aware of is that Part D drug plans have to have a medication therapy management program. These programs are designed to help beneficiaries who have multiple chronic diseases and who take multiple prescription drugs to improve their health. The intention is to reduce the cost of the medications for these individuals. This is done by having health care professionals identify Medicare beneficiaries who are already enrolled in their Part D drug plan and who might benefit from such a program. Physicians may be involved in this process, but much of the work is done by registered nurses and pharmacists.

Beginning in 2010, you will be routinely enrolled in this program if you meet the criteria, which are shown below. You can then opt out of the program whenever you wish. These professionals will then take an intervention, which means trying to improve your health by changing the medicines you take and/or by adjusting the doses you receive. The intervention will be an annual "comprehensive medical review" of all of your prescription and non-prescription medicines, dietary supplements, and herbal remedies. Furthermore, you must be offered a person-to-person consultation (typically by phone) and a written take-away, which means an action plan or a recommendation for further education.

Each Part D plan has its own criteria to be enrolled in the medication therapy management program. The requirements set by Medicare states that the beneficiary has to —

- have three chronic diseases,

- be taking eight or more prescriptions, and

- be incurring $3,000 worth of Part D covered drugs a year.

In all likelihood, your plan's criteria will be lower than these maximums, so you may be enrolled in one of these programs even if you are taking only six prescriptions. Check the guidelines set out by your plan to determine whether you are eligible.

7. Part D: Details of Coverage

Part D covers a majority of prescription drugs, but not all drugs are covered. The following are the drug categories that are *not* covered:

- Barbiturates and benzodiazepines (often used for seizure and anxiety control)

- Cold and cough symptomatic relief medications

- Drugs for cosmetic purposes, including for hair growth

- Fertility drugs

- Vitamins and minerals, even if prescribed (with the exception of prenatal vitamins and fluorides, which are covered)

- Drugs for weight gain, weight loss, or anorexia (even those prescribed to treat morbid obesity)

- Erectile or sexual dysfunction medicines

There is some confusion about the coverage of erectile dysfunction drugs. (The three main drugs are Viagra®, Cialis®, and Levitra®.) These drugs are covered under Part D only if used to treat a non-erectile dysfunction condition specifically approved by the Food and Drug Administration. It may be that your drug plan covers these drugs in its supplemental benefit package.

Plans must cover all, or substantially all, drugs in the following categories:

- Anti-cancer

- Anticonvulsants

- Antidepressants

- Antipsychotics

- Antiretrovirals (usually used in AIDS therapy)

- Immunosuppressants

- Insulin, and the supplies necessary to administer it (this includes inhalable insulin and the inhalation chamber used to ingest it)

Note that prescription smoking cessation agents are also covered.

7.1 How Part D works with Part A and Part B

You should know that drugs that are covered by Medicare Part A or Part B are not covered by Part D. This should concern you only if you get one of those drugs covered ordinarily by Part B (see Chapter 4, section **2.21**, for more information) and you don't have Part B. In these situations, Part D will not cover the drug even though it may be a prescription medicine.

One exception exists in the very rare case that a Part A beneficiary runs out of his or her Part A inpatient days. If this is your situation, and you have Part D, drugs that your Part D drug plan would ordinarily cover must now be covered for you even though you remain in the facility. In other words, supposing your Part A benefits are exhausted, Part D now has to cover your drugs because Part A has ceased to do so. Drug plans are responsible to insure that proper arrangements are made for the drugs to be supplied through a pharmacy to you, the beneficiary, while you are an inpatient.

7.1a Vaccines

One oddity of the drug benefit surrounds the administration of vaccines. While Part D plans must cover all commercially available vaccines, the issue is paying for the administration of the vaccine. (You have to pay extra to get stuck with a needle!) Your Part D plan has to help with the cost. Remember that vaccines covered by Part B are not involved in this, because if a drug is covered under Part B, Part D can't cover it. If you need a vaccine that you can't get under Part B, you can call your drug plan and ask how it will handle paying for its share of the vaccine and the administration.

Most states allow pharmacists to administer vaccines, and if your drug plan has a network pharmacy that will do this, the simplest thing to do is to get your doctor to call in a prescription for the vaccine, and get the vaccine administered by the pharmacist. The pharmacy will bill your plan directly for its share of the cost of both the vaccine and the administration, and will bill you for the applicable deductible and coinsurance.

You can get the pharmacy to deliver the vaccine to your doctor's office. The pharmacy will make you pay the applicable Part D coinsurance and/or deductible for the vaccine. Typically the doctor's office will then administer it, and charge you the full cost for the administration. You'll have to send in a paper claim to your Part D plan to be compensated for its share of the administration fee.

There is another variation, such as the doctor may already have the vaccine, and make you pay for it and the administration, and you then submit a claim for both items to your plan. You will have to call your plan and your doctor's office to figure out how to proceed.

7.1b Nursing home stays

If you are a Medicare beneficiary, and your stay in a Skilled Nursing Facility is covered by Medicare, your Part A — not your Part D — will pay for all your medicines.

If you are in a nursing home and are a dual Medicare and Medicaid beneficiary, your Medicare Part D will pay for your medicines and you will not have to pay anything for them. If you are not dually entitled, but are a Medicare beneficiary who has Part D, your drug plan will pay for your prescription medicines even when you are in a nursing home.

You should know that nursing homes have to deal with a long-term care pharmacy, and it's helpful if your drug plan works with the particular long-term care pharmacy that deals with your nursing home. If it does not, you should consider changing to a drug plan that does, but only if that plan will cover the medicines you need. Any Part D beneficiary staying in a nursing home can switch drug plans once a month. This is to help ensure your Part D plan covers the medicines you need.

7.2 If you have Medicaid

If you are a Medicaid beneficiary, and you are also entitled to Medicare (e.g., you reach age 65), almost all of your prescription drugs will now be covered by Medicare instead of Medicaid. You will get continuous prescription drug coverage from Medicare, it will pay your premium, and you pay very little or nothing for each prescription, although you may actually pay slightly more than you are currently paying under Medicaid. (If you are fully eligible for both programs and live in a nursing home, you will pay nothing for your Part D drugs.)

When you get your Medicare, you will automatically be enrolled in a Part D plan if you did not already choose one. If you want to be in another plan, you can change drug plans any month you want to. An exception to this is that if the Centers for Medicare & Medicaid Services know you have retiree coverage, it will not automatically enroll you in Part D, but instead send you a notice telling you that you have the option of enrolling but that you should contact your retiree coverage plan's benefits advisor to go over the situation before you do anything. This is because if you enroll in Part D, you may lose all or part of your retiree coverage, your spouse may lose his or hers, and you may never be able to get it back.

Finally, note that some drugs were covered under Medicaid may not be covered under Medicare. In some states Medicaid will continue to cover these medicines. Your Medicaid contact in your locality, county, or state will be able to clarify this.

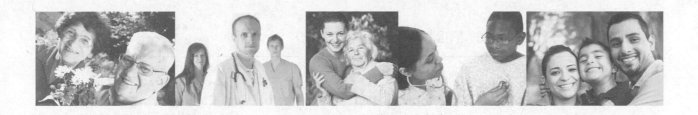

7

Part D: Extra Help with Your Prescription Drug Benefit

If you have low income and limited assets, you may be eligible for Extra Help with your Part D drug benefit. This means that the Medicare program will pay part or all of your monthly Part D premium; it will reduce and maybe even eliminate your annual deductible; and it will limit, even through the coverage gap, what you pay for any drug to either a small dollar amount or to 15 percent of the price of the drug. This Extra Help feature of Medicare Part D has been important since its inception as a way to help low-income and low-resource beneficiaries with the high cost of prescription drugs.

1. What Extra Help Covers

Your entitlement to other programs, whether or not you are in a nursing home, your income level, and the extent of your resources all determine how Extra Help assists in paying for your Part D premiums, deductibles, and co-payments. It's easier to understand all this by referring to Table 10, which lays this out in some detail. Note that this uses 2009 figures as 2010 information was not yet available at the time of printing this book. Let's go down

through the following table row-by-row so you can get a better idea of just how much help you'll get with Extra Help.

As the first row shows, if you have Medicaid, Extra Help will pay all of your Part D monthly premium. You won't have to meet any annual deductible, and your co-payment for any prescription will never be more than $6.00. Finally, once you are past the coverage gap (i.e., the donut hole) and into the catastrophic level, you will pay nothing for any prescription.

The second row shows that if your state helps pay your Medicare Part B premiums (i.e., you are in the Medicare Savings Program discussed in Chapter 1 as a Qualified Medicare Beneficiary, a Specified Low-Income Medicare Beneficiary, or as a Qualified Individual), or if you get Supplemental Security Income (SSI), extra help will pay all of your Part D monthly premium. You won't have to meet any annual deductible, and your co-payment for any prescription will never be more than $6.00. Finally, once you are past the coverage gap (i.e., the donut hole) and into the catastrophic level, you will pay nothing for any prescription.

TABLE 10
SIMPLIFIED EXTRA HELP FOR 2009 (FOR LOWER 48 STATES ONLY)

Your Status	Percent of Monthly Premium Paid for by Extra Help	Your Annual Deductible	Your Cost or Co-payment for Each Prescription	Your Cost for Each Prescription (after the Coverage Gap Stage)
		Will not exceed		
You have Medicaid	100%	$0	$6.00	$0
Your state helps you pay your Medicare premiums or you get Social Security Income	100%	$0	$6.00	$0
Your income is less than $14,621 (individual) or $19,670 (couple) and your resources are at or less than $6,600 (individual) or $9,910 (couple)	100%	$0	$6.00	$0
Your income is less than $16,245 (individual) or $21,855 (couple) and your resources are at or less than $11,010 (individual) or $22,010 (couple)	from 100% down to 25%	$60	15%	$6.00

The third row shows that if your annual income is below $14,621 for an individual or $19,670 for a couple, and your resources are at or less than $6,600 for an individual or $9,910 for a couple, then Extra Help will pay all of your monthly Part D premium. You won't have to meet any annual deductible, and your co-payment for any prescription will never be more than $6. Finally, once you are past the coverage gap (i.e., donut hole) and into the catastrophic level, you will pay nothing for any prescription.

The fourth row covers those whose income is less than $16,245 for an individual or $21,855 for a couple and whose resources are at or less than $11,010 for an individual or $22,010 for a couple. Extra Help will pay either all of your monthly Part D premium, three-quarters of it, half of it, or a quarter of it, depending on the exact amount of your income and resources. No matter how much of your premium it pays, your annual deductible will never be more than $60. You will never have to pay more than a 15 percent co-payment for a prescription. Finally, once you are past the coverage gap (i.e., the donut hole) and into the catastrophic level, you will never pay more than $6 for any prescription.

For more exact information, as well as the specific limits for Alaska and Hawaii, see Extra Help Extended Tables on the CD.

Sometimes you will see similar information to that in Table 10, but the annual income levels are $2,880 higher, and the resources levels are higher by $1,500 for an individual and $3,000 for a couple. That information is not incorrect; it recognizes that these amounts are automatically disregarded in making your income and resource calculations. The amounts shown here are the same that the Social Security Administration will use in taking all of your income and resources into account, and then determining what does and does not count toward Extra Help. The important point is that if your income and resources are anywhere near the ones shown in Table 10 or the Extra Help Extended Tables on the CD, you should apply for Extra Help. This is especially true because of the many rules and disregards that reduce your actual income and resources when figuring out if you qualify for Extra Help.

Table 10 and the Extra Help Extended Tables on the CD have information for 2009. The pertinent information for 2010 will not be known until well into 2010, so it's best to keep this information consistent with one year, even though we know, for example, that the $6 shown in Table 10 will change to $6.30 in 2010, but we do not know what the new income and resource levels will be.

Note: Where Table 10 and the Extra Help Extended Tables on the CD show a percentage or a dollar amount for your co-payment, you will pay the lower of this percent or amount, or of what you would otherwise have to pay for your drug. For example, if you buy a preferred drug and your Part D plan's rules say you have to pay a co-payment of $10 for this drug, it prices at $100 while the Extra Help rules say you pay 15 percent, then you pay only this $10, and not 15 percent of $100.

2. Automatic Qualification

Some Medicare beneficiaries will automatically be put into the extra help program. Specifically, those people who have Medicaid when they become eligible for Medicare, and those people who are receiving Supplemental Security Income and become eligible for Medicare, will automatically be put into Extra Help. The Supplemental Security Income program is where you get a monthly check or payment from the federal government because you have limited income and resources and are aged, blind, or disabled. These payments are not the same thing as Social Security payments.

If you qualify for the Medicare Savings Program (see section **8.3** in Chapter 1) in which your state pays your Part B premiums, you will also meet the criteria for extra help. Remember that this is a state program, and you need to apply to your state for this. Note that each state's income and resource requirements for automatic qualifications are much stricter than the extra help program — that is, the income limits are much lower — so it is harder to qualify for this. If you do qualify, your state will then make this information available to Medicare so you can also qualify for Extra Help, which is a federal, not a state, program. This underscores the need for you to apply for the assistance your state will give you with Part B, as you will also be applying for Extra Help.

Even if you apply to your state for automatic coverage, you should also apply to Social Security for Extra Help as explained in the next section, because the criteria for getting it are much easier than for state programs. This way, if your request for Part B help is not approved by your state, you may still be able to get Extra Help with Part D.

3. Applying for Extra Help

In order to apply for Extra Help, call the Social Security Administration and ask for an application or go online and apply. You should not submit any documentation or supporting evidence with your application form. If Social Security needs anything more, it will call or write you. It may become necessary for you to visit one of its local offices, but this is not a usual occurrence.

The Social Security Administration will make its decision based on the income and resource limits which are in effect at the time it makes its decision. The income limits change every year and they are based on what is called the official Federal Poverty Limits (FPL). These are simply annual income figures, which the federal government publishes and which are used to establish people's eligibility for various federal and state programs. For example, the FPL for a one-person family in 2009 is $10,830. If you want to qualify for a program, let's say energy assistance program, and it requires you to have an income of 100 percent of the FPL or less, then your annual income has to be $10,830 or less for you to qualify. The updated income amounts for a given year are established by the federal government in January of that same year. As it takes time to reprogram the various systems used to make determinations, the old year's income guides are used in the early months of the new year.

Note that the government establishes different limits depending on how many people are in a household — the more people, the higher the FPL. Note that the FPLs are not the same for the whole country; they are higher for the states of Alaska and Hawaii because it costs so much more to live in those places. As indicated earlier, the most generous levels of Extra Help are available to those whose incomes are at or less than the basic or 100 percent FPL annual income amounts. These are shown in Table 11.

To qualify at all for the Extra Help program, your income can be up to one-and-a-half times (150 percent) the FPL. Because of this threshold, Table 12 shows what the 150 percent FPL annual income amounts are for 2009. You can use this information based on where you live and how large your family is to see if you could qualify for extra help.

To repeat an important point, because of the ways income is counted, even if your income is somewhat higher than these amounts, you should apply for Extra Help. Section 4.1 will give you more information about what does and does not count as income.

The resource limits also change every year and are updated using an Urban Consumer Price Index. Unlike the income limits, these are the same throughout the nation. These go into effect January 1 of each calendar year; there is no delay in applying them in the new year. In section 4.2 there is more information about what do and do not count as resources.

After you have applied for Extra Help, you will get a formal notice from the Social Security Administration telling you if you qualify. If you do, you will also get the Green Letter from the Centers for Medicaid & Medicare Services (CMS Publication No. 11186), which will tell you to enroll in a Part D plan (or Medicare will go ahead and enroll you in one). As mentioned in Chapter 6, you should pick your plan depending on your prescriptions and the premium amount.

4. Income and Resources for Extra Help Purposes

Once you apply to the Social Security Administration for Extra Help as a person with low income and low resources, it will use the information in your application, as well as other information it has on hand (e.g., the amount of your Social Security check, or the amounts of the wages you earn or self-employment income you make, both of which are posted to its records), to determine what your income and resources are for Extra Help purposes. It may need to get more information from you before it makes its decision.

You need to accurately and completely fill in your application. The kinds of income and resources Social Security will count in determining whether you qualify for Extra Help along with some of the special rules it uses in making these decisions are discussed in the next few sections. As you will see, what does and doesn't get counted can become complicated, and so if you are anywhere near the limits discussed earlier, you are always much better off applying and getting turned down than not applying at all.

4.1 Income

Income is looked at very differently depending on whether it is earned or unearned. The following two sections will help you understand the difference between these two types of income.

4.1a Unearned income

Unearned income that is counted typically includes pensions, annuities, and disability payments, such as the following:

- Social Security benefits of all kinds
- Railroad Retirement Board benefits of all kinds
- Veterans Benefits
- Workers' Compensation
- Pensions from a company, union, or government entity

Note that if any Medicare premium (normally your Part B and maybe your Part D premium) is being deducted from your monthly payments, these have to be added back in to get your total benefit amount.

The following periodic and one-time payments you receive are also counted:

- Alimony and support payments
- Prizes
- Awards
- Net (not gross) rental income

TABLE 11
100 PERCENT OF THE FEDERAL POVERTY LIMIT (2009)

	Lower 48 States	Alaska	Hawaii
Individual	$10,830	$13,530	$12,460
Couple	$14,570	$18,210	$16,760
Each additional family member	$3,740	$4,680	$4,300

TABLE 12
150 PERCENT OF THE FEDERAL POVERTY LIMIT (2009)

	Lower 48 States	Alaska	Hawaii
Individual	$16,245	$20,295	$18,690
Couple	$21,855	$27,315	$25,140
Each additional family member	$5,610	$7,020	$6,450

Certain infrequent and irregular payments of unearned income have exclusions of up to $60 in any calendar quarter. For example, if your bank sends you a one-time bonus of $25 because you kept your checking account with the bank for a full year, this would be excluded.

In determining the total amount of your unearned income that counts toward the Extra Help income limits, the first $20 of any unearned income in a month is excluded no matter what. If the $20 is not all used here, the remainder of the exclusion applies to earned income.

Another form of unearned income is in-kind support and maintenance. This generally consists of the help you get, usually from a family member or possibly an organization such as a church, with living expenses and arrangements, including:

- Shelter, that is, help with mortgage, taxes, rent, and utilities (e.g., electricity, water, garbage, sewer)
- Food

For applications filed for extra help in 2010, none of this type of income will count toward income for Extra Help purposes. So if you were once turned down because of receiving unearned income, apply again.

4.1b Earned income

Earned income is income from wages and self-employment. Note that all of these are included in determining your income for Extra Help purposes.

- Salary and wages (before deductions)
- Tips
- Self-employment income (net only)
- Share of profits or losses from a partnership

- Commissions
- Bonuses

It is very important for you to know that there are huge exclusions about earned income. The first $65 each month is excluded, and half of the remaining amount is also excluded. For example, if you made $500 one month, your income for extra help purposes is only $217.50 ($500 - $65 = $435, and $435 divided by 2 = $217.50).

In addition, certain payments of infrequent and irregular earned income have exclusions of up to $30 in a calendar quarter. For example, perhaps you worked very briefly one quarter and earned a total of $200 in the whole three months. Only $170 of this would be counted toward your income for Extra Help purposes.

4.1c Exclusions from income

The following are excluded from income:

- Jurors' fees
- Hobby income
- Income tax refunds
- Rebates
- Dividends
- Interest
- Medical services
- Social services
- Food stamps
- Energy assistance programs (e.g., heating and cooling)
- Federal housing subsidies
- Economic stimulus payments

Interest income or dividends are excluded from Extra Help purposes because the investments that generate these will be considered under resources. Some information you may find online or from other sources will tell you that these items count as income, but that is incorrect.

4.2 Resources and assets

As with income, you have to determine what your assets or resources are to see if you qualify for Extra Help. You also need to understand that the level of help you get, if any, also depends on how much resources or assets you have.

4.2a Cash and equivalents

Generally cash equivalent is something that could be converted into cash in 20 days. The following count as cash and equivalents:

- Checking account balances
- Savings accounts
- Certificates of deposit
- Stocks
- Bonds
- US Savings Bonds
- Mutual funds
- IRAs of all types
- Roth accounts
- Promissory notes you hold
- Trusts; that is, revocable trusts and those where the applicant for Extra Help can direct the use of the funds (other trust arrangements may not count)

4.2b Exclusions to resources

Resources or assets do not include the following:

- Your home and the lot, property, farm, or ranch on which it is located, or any other buildings on the same property

- Vehicles or any transportation device (e.g., snowmobile)
- Household goods, furniture, and appliances
- Personal effects (e.g., clothing, jewelry, electronics)
- Life insurance policies
- Any business or nonbusiness property essential to your self-support (e.g., a rental property which produces earnings vital to your self-support)
- A straight $1,500 of any resource if you deem that you will use it for burial purposes ($3,000 for a couple) whether or not you have any other burial arrangements
- A burial policy (i.e., a policy that pays only the actual costs of final arrangements and burial) no matter what its value
- Burial plots or spaces
- Certain nonbusiness property used to produce goods or services essential to your self-support (e.g., a plot of land you use to grow the food you eat)

Just to show you how convoluted the rules can be, it was noted earlier that US Savings Bonds do count as resources; however, they do not count if the bonds you hold happen to be in the non-redemption period (i.e., usually the first 6 or 12 months of ownership, depending on the type or series of the particular bond you hold). This is because you cannot convert them into cash in that period.

If you own a paper US Savings Bond (but not the kind in electronic form) and you are unable to physically possess it (maybe you have misplaced it and after searching high and low you haven't yet been able to find it), it does not count as a resource as you can't readily redeem it if you don't physically have it.

5. Special Family Situations

You should understand that you are considered married only if you are legally married and are living with your spouse. If you are legally separated, or if you don't live together, you are considered single for Extra Help purposes. However, if you are legally married and are living with your spouse, even if only one of you applies for this (it may be that your spouse is not yet entitled to Medicare), the Social Security Administration will look at the income and resources of both of you.

Income limits are higher for those who pay more than half of the living expenses of dependent family members who live with them. Perhaps you have an aged parent living with you and you support this parent. This raises the amount of income you can get and still qualify for Extra Help. Again, because of the complexity of these rules, if your income and/or resources are anywhere near the amounts in Table 10 or the Extra Help Extended Tables on the CD, or if you have a special family situation, you should apply.

6. Special Circumstances in Qualifying for Extra Help

The Centers for Medicare & Medicaid Services have insisted that Part D drug plans accept evidence presented by beneficiaries or their representatives that they are entitled to Extra Help, or even a change in their Extra Help status. For example, you may have recently been entitled to Medicaid and now qualify for Extra Help, but somehow this determination by your state's Medicaid agency has not been transmitted to the Centers for Medicare & Medicaid Services. In this situation, you can supply evidence of your Medicaid eligibility to your Part D plan and, in turn, the plan has to report this to the Medicare people and put you on as a Medicaid eligible in its Part D system.

Perhaps you already had Medicaid and now you go into a nursing home, which changes the level of assistance you receive from Extra Help. Again, if you supply evidence of this to your Part D plan, it is supposed to make sure you are put at the correct level of Extra Help. The Centers for Medicare & Medicaid Services have not specified all the types of evidence Part D plans have to accept, so you will need to contact your plan to discuss your situation, but items such as entitlement letters from your state or county, Medicaid eligibility cards, or printouts from the Medicaid eligibility system qualify.

Also, Medicare advises that if you have to get a prescription filled before you get your enrollment card from a drug plan, bring all the information and letters you have about you getting Extra Help and joining a plan, as well as photo identification and your red, white, and blue Medicare card to the drugstore. The pharmacist may be able to confirm your enrollment and dispense your prescription. If not, and you purchase any medicines, save your receipts and submit them to your drug plan for reimbursement. Even if you do not have Extra Help, the same general advice applies to you.

7. Premium Limits for Extra Help Beneficiaries

Every year the Medicare actuaries have to calculate a sort of mid-point premium amount for each state, and that is the most that Medicare will pay for an Extra Help premium. In other words, Medicare will not pay its full share of the higher-end premiums in which Extra Help is involved. These state-by-state amounts are sometimes called premium benchmarks.

Table 13 shows the number of Part D plans that Medicare will pay its full share of the premium, and the highest premium it will pay in full. Note that these numbers and amounts will change every year.

TABLE 13
EXTRA HELP PREMIUM BENCHMARK INFORMATION (2010)

State	No. of Plans with Premiums at or below Cut-off	Low-Income Subsidy Premium	State	No. of Plans with Premiums at or below Cut-off	Low-Income Subsidy Premium
Alabama	11	$30.70	Nebraska	13	$37.50
Alaska	8	$38.00	Nevada	7	$27.30
Arizona	7	$27.30	New Hampshire	6	$27.00
Arkansas	15	$28.50	New Jersey	7	$35.00
California	8	$29.00	New Mexico	11	$21.40
Colorado	8	$31.00	New York	11	$33.30
Connecticut	14	$34.60	North Carolina	10	$34.90
Delaware	13	$33.70	North Dakota	13	$37.50
District of Columbia	13	$33.70	Ohio	7	$30.50
Florida	8	$27.40	Oklahoma	11	$32.30
Georgia	9	$29.60	Oregon	13	$35.60
Hawaii	10	$25.60	Pennsylvania	15	$32.10
Idaho	12	$10.90	Puerto Rico	N/A	
Illinois	12	$31.60	Rhode Island	14	$34.60
Indiana	13	$35.70	South Carolina	17	$35.00
Iowa	13	$37.50	South Dakota	13	$37.50
Kansas	12	$35.80	Tennessee	11	$30.70
Kentucky	13	$35.70	Texas	11	$27.50
Louisiana	13	$31.30	Utah	12	$40.90
Maine	6	$27.00	Vermont	14	$34.60
Maryland	13	$33.70	Virginia	14	$34.10
Massachusetts	14	$34.60	Virgin Islands	N/A	
Michigan	11	$34.90	Washington	13	$33.60
Minnesota	13	$37.50	West Virginia	15	$32.10
Mississippi	13	$33.00	Wisconsin	15	$38.20
Missouri	17	$40.00	Wyoming	13	$37.50
Montana	13	$37.50			

*Note: Puerto Rico and the Virgin Islands cannot participate in the Low-Income Subsidy (Extra Help) program.

Extra Help is available to residents of the 50 states and the District of Columbia. It is not available to residents of the Commonwealth of Puerto Rico and the Territory of the Virgin Islands. However, low-income and low-resource beneficiaries in these two jurisdictions may be able to get help from their Medicaid offices; the phone numbers for Medicaid are in the Resources section on the CD.

Please understand that Medicare will pay up to its share of the amounts listed in Table 13. If your premium is subsidized in full, that is, Medicare is supposed to pay 100 percent of it, and your plan's premium is $40 in a state where the benchmark or maximum is $30, Medicare will pay $30, and you will pay $10. If Medicare subsidizes 50 percent of your premium, it will pay $15 (half of the limit of $30) and you will have to pay $25.

If Medicare automatically signs you up for a Part D drug plan, it will sign you up for one less than the limit. It may be that from one year to the next your plan raises its premium so that Medicare no longer pays it in full. If this happens, you will be notified of this and given the opportunity to choose another plan. This notification is ordinarily done in the Blue Letter (CMS Publication 11209).

It may be that, given the specific drugs you take, you would be better off in a plan in which you have to pay more of the premium than usual. This will happen if no plan in which Medicare pays its full share of the premium has all the specific drugs you take, that is, if your drugs aren't on its formulary. You should call Medicare or a counselor at your State Health Insurance Assistance Program (SHIP) to find the best plan for you.

You should also understand that for those of you who choose to sign up for a Medicare Advantage or managed care plan that includes your prescription drug Part D benefit, you are also subject to this limit. It is for this reason that Medicare gives you information about what portion of a Medicare Advantage Plan's premium is for the Part D drug benefit, and what portion is for all its other benefits. You can find this information on the Medicare website.

8. Changes and Redeterminations to Your Extra Help Status

If you are determined to be eligible for Extra Help, this may change over time; it is possible that you will lose your Extra Help. Your eligibility at a particular level may increase or decrease depending on your circumstances. Some of these changes will be made as a result of something you report to the Social Security Administration; in other cases they will be made because the agency will get information about you. In addition, the Social Security Administration has operations in place that will periodically check on beneficiaries' eligibility for Extra Help and their level of subsidy.

Medicare beneficiaries receiving Extra Help do not have to report any events to the Social Security Administration on account of their involvement in this particular program. However, changes that are reported to Social Security or Medicare will be forwarded to the extra help databases, and action will be taken to redetermine your benefit. For example, if you are receiving Extra Help, and you also report the death of a spouse to the Social Security Administration because your spouse received a Social Security check, that information will also be processed by the Extra Help program.

You should also be aware that increases or decreases in your resources and income levels will not change your Extra Help subsidy when they occur, but that once you get Extra Help, you keep it for that whole calendar year, and you keep it at the particular level that you first got it at. That can be good for you if your income or resources increase; for example, a relative bequeaths you $50,000. That puts you higher than the resource limit, but your Extra Help will continue for that year. Another example is that your income decreases, maybe because a company that is paying you a modest pension goes out of business and you no longer get your pension. You can't change your subsidy level and have Extra Help pay more of your drug costs until the next year.

8.1 Subsidy changing events

There are some events, which are called subsidy changing events, that cause the Social Security Administration to immediately take action to change your Extra Help status. These events all involve marital situations such as:

- You marry and begin living with your new spouse.

- The spouse you live with dies.

- You and the spouse you live with are divorced, separated, or your marriage is annulled.

- You and your separated spouse begin living together again.

If something happens that will lessen your Extra Help subsidy, you should not report it because you have no requirement as an Extra Help beneficiary to do so. If something happens that would increase your subsidy, you should report it because you will benefit by doing so. For example, suppose you and your spouse are getting the level of Extra Help that pays 50 percent of your Part D premium, and you separate. As a result of your separation, your income level drops from $21,500 as a couple to $14,800 as an individual. You would now qualify for 100 percent of your premium to be paid. In this case, you should report this change right away. However,

if you get back together, you shouldn't report that, as your subsidy level will be reduced. Wait until the redetermination process gets around to you as you are not required to report these events for Extra Help purposes (although you may be required to for other purposes).

8.2 Redeterminations

The redetermination process merely means that the Social Security Administration will periodically send out letters to review beneficiaries' continued eligibility for Extra Help. These letters are usually mailed in August.

You should expect to get this letter and a redetermination form if you first became eligible anytime beginning in May of the prior year through April of the current year. The agency will also look through its files and ask for a redetermination in other cases where it thinks there may be some likelihood of change.

You will get the form immediately if you report a subsidy changing event, or if you report a nonsubsidy changing event after the Social Security Administration makes its general mailing in August.

8.3 Extra Help notices

It's the Centers for Medicare & Medicaid Services (CMS) that actually sends out notices about your Extra Help. These letters are color coded so when you call CMS about them, you'll be asked what color the letter is and this will help CMS know exactly which one you received.

You may not get any of the following letters because your situation will remain stable in the year ahead. However, all beneficiaries who have Extra Help will get, along with their Annual Notice of Change from their drug plan, a rider telling them how their Extra Help will work with their plan in the coming year. This will help beneficiaries to confirm their status in the coming calendar year.

8.3a Gray letter

The gray letter is sent out in September, and it will tell you that you have lost your deemed status for Extra Help as you no longer get Supplemental Security Income (SSI), or Medicaid, or your state no longer helps with your Medicare premiums (i.e., you are no longer in the Medicare Savings Program). However, the Gray Letter spells out the requirements for non-deemed status for extra help, and invites you to apply to the Social Security Administration if you think you meet the income and resources levels.

8.3b Orange letter

The orange letter tells you that you will continue to get Extra Help, but at a level that is slightly different than you have been getting. This letter is sent out in October, but the effective date of the change is not until January 1. Although this entails only a small change in your level of co-payments, the letter does tell you to call the Centers for Medicare & Medicaid Services if you don't understand it or if you think the decision is wrong.

8.3c Tan letter

The tan letter will tell you that, beginning the next calendar year, the government will no longer pay the full premium of the drug plan you are currently in. Or, if you are a partial subsidy beneficiary in which you have to pay 25 percent, 50 percent, or 75 percent of your plan's Part D premium, that it will no longer pay its full share as of January. This will happen because the drug plan you are in is raising its premium higher than the amount the government will pay in full.

The best thing to do is to search for a plan that will cover all of your prescriptions and which has a premium below the benchmark for your state. The tan letter will list the specific plans in your state for which the government will pay its full share of the whole premium.

8.3d Blue letter

The blue letter tells you that you will be reassigned to a new drug plan beginning January 1. This reassignment will be made because you are in a plan that is leaving the Part D program, or you had been automatically enrolled into a plan with a premium that is rising to the extent that the government will no longer pay its full share.

You can either let the Medicare computer assign you to a new plan, or you can contact your local State Health Insurance Assistance Program (SHIP) with a complete list of all your prescriptions, and have SHIP help you look for a plan that will be best for you in the next year.

9. Appealing an Extra Help Decision

Once Social Security makes a decision on your application (this typically takes several weeks) it may send you an award notice saying you are eligible for Extra Help, and for how much, and telling you that you need to enroll in a drug plan. Or, it may send you a pre-decisional notice indicating that it plans to deny your application and the reason for that. If you get one of these, it's because Social Security thinks that you do not meet the requirements for Extra Help and you may be asked to explain further any issues that preclude your successful application.

Whether or not you respond to this notice (you are supposed to respond within ten calendar days), Social Security will subsequently send you a formal award or denial notice. You can appeal this notice (but not the pre-decisional one). The award or denial notice will have two attachments; one showing how Social Security figured your "income," and the other, your "resources."

The tricky thing here is that you will obviously know to appeal a denial notice. However, there are many levels of Extra Help, and it's not easy to tell if you are getting all the Extra Help you should. Your will have to carefully compare the income and resources decisions accompanying your award notice to the information in Table 10 or by using the Extra Help Extended Tables on the CD to decide if you are getting all the help you should.

If you believe that Social Security has improperly denied your application, or, even if you get an award notice, that Social Security is not giving you as much Extra Help as you believe you should get, you can formally appeal the decision.

Unlike the appeal process for almost all Social Security and Medicare related matters, the one for Extra Help is extremely abbreviated. You only get one chance to make your appeal administratively, and then you have to go all the way to a civil suit in a US District Court.

You can appeal by calling Social Security and asking for an appeal; no signature is necessary.

Or, you may file an Appeal of Determination for Help with Medicare Prescription Drug Costs (Form SSA-1021), downloadable from the Social Security website.

If you are granted a hearing for your appeal, you need to carefully consider what additional information or documentation you need to present to Social Security, and get it to Social Security. Make sure you can very clearly articulate the reasons you should prevail in the hearing, probably by writing this out. This is important because it is a one-shot process, and you really need to be prepared before you go through with the hearing.

You will then get either an award notice (or a revised one, if your appeal for a different level of help was approved) or a letter explaining why Social Security thinks its decision was correct.

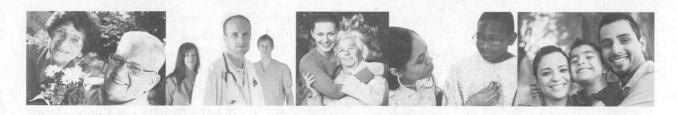

8

Part C: Medicare Advantage Plans and Enrollment Requirements

An increasing number of beneficiaries are choosing Medicare Advantage, which is the program's name for managed care. It's also sometimes called Part C.

To join a Medicare managed care organization, you have to have Medicare Part A and Part B. Once you join, you essentially have to adhere to your managed care organization's rules about what care you get, from which physician and provider you get it, and when and how much care you get. You usually have to pay your plan a monthly premium, in addition to the Part B premium that you already pay. Because you are beholden to your plan for your medical care, the Medicare program has some powerful rights you can exercise to ensure that you get good care.

For beneficiaries who do not carry a health insurance plan of some sort into their Medicare years, or who want to avoid paying for a Medigap policy, joining a Medicare Advantage program should be strongly considered.

This chapter will help you understand the different types of Medicare Advantage Plans and the enrollment requirements.

1. Types of Medicare Advantage Plans

It is helpful to know what types of Medicare Advantage Plans are available to you so you can decide whether or not you want to go into managed care.

1.1 Point-of-Service (POS) option

Many Medicare Advantage Plans offer a Point-of-Service (POS) benefit option. This option allows beneficiaries to go outside the plan network without obtaining a special authorization to get services. Some plans offer this to all their beneficiary members, and others offer it as an option. If it is offered as an option, you have to pay a higher monthly premium for it. Usually you will incur higher costs for such point-of-service care. For example, you might be charged a co-payment of $25 to see a doctor of your own choice rather than $10 if you went to the same kind of doctor in your plan's network. Some plans may limit the services you can obtain this way, or how often you can do this.

You should be aware of a couple of cautions when using POS. One is to be sure the doctor or provider you go to out-of-network agrees to take your Medicare Advantage Plan's payment for your treatment, and he or she knows the correct amount of the co-payment he or she should charge you. The other is that, if you begin using this option a lot, you may want to think about whether you are in the right kind of Medicare Advantage Plan for you. Would you be better off with a different plan that includes all or most of the out-of-network providers you are going to?

1.2 Religious Fraternal Benefit plans

The Religious Fraternal Benefit plans are Medicare Advantage Plans of any type that are offered by a religious or fraternal benefit society or organization recognized by the Internal Revenue Service (IRS), and which limit enrollment exclusively to members of that society or organization.

1.3 Health Maintenance Organizations (HMO)

The Health Maintenance Organizations (HMO) are Medicare Advantage coordinated care plans that generally restrict beneficiaries to receiving services from their specific network of providers. Sometimes these providers are employees of the HMO. Sometimes they have agreements with the HMO to be a provider.

Typically, a beneficiary needs a referral from a primary care physician to get most services. Some services will require a prior authorization from the organization itself. Beneficiaries can usually get their Part D prescription drug coverage through their HMO.

1.4 Provider Sponsored Organizations (PSO)

Provider Sponsored Organizations (PSO) are Medicare Advantage coordinated care plans that are organized and operated by one or more health-care providers, who typically render most of the care, although usually there are also affiliated or contracted providers in their network.

Typically, as with other coordinated care plans, you need a referral and, at times, a prior authorization from the organization itself. You can usually get your Part D prescription drug coverage through your PSO.

1.5 Preferred Provider Organizations (PPO)

Preferred Provider Organizations (PPO) are Medicare Advantage coordinated care plans with a network of providers that have contracted with the plan to deliver services to members. Although these outfits are usually not as strict as the other coordinated care plans previously mentioned, you might need a referral or prior authorization to get services. You can usually get your Part D prescription drug coverage through your PPO.

Note that Medicare makes a big distinction between regional and local PPOs. Medicare has divided the 50 states into 26 PPO regions (Puerto Rico is not included). Many of these regions include only one state, such as California; while others have two, such as New Hampshire and Maine; and at least one has seven states, which are South Dakota, North Dakota, Iowa, Minnesota, Montana, Nebraska, and Wyoming. If a new PPO wants to do business in one of these areas, it has to offer a plan that covers the whole region and it has to offer the same premium and benefits throughout the entire area.

In addition, you may find yourself in an area where other plans have high premiums, but because the regional PPO plans must have a uniform premium, you might be able to find one of these with a lower premium than similar plans in your area.

There is one Medicare requirement for regional PPOs that local PPOs do not have to meet, but which is very valuable for beneficiaries. Regional PPOs must have an annual out-of-pocket maximum; that is, they have to establish a money amount beyond which they will pay for everything that is covered. (Many people call these catastrophic caps or limits.) Sometimes these amounts are separate as to whether or not you get the services from preferred providers (in-network) or out-of-network. For example, a regional PPO may have an in-network limit of $3,000 and an out-of-network limit of $4,000. It will pay, once you have spent $3,000 on in-network services, anything higher than that for covered in-network services. Separately, after you have spent $4,000 on out-of-network, it will pay 100 percent of what is covered after that. The PPO may have a combined maximum of $5,000; so after you have spent a total of $5,000 on services (whether in-network or out-of-network) it picks up the whole tab for covered services. If possible, look for one with a combined limitation on your out-of-pocket expenses.

You should be aware that many local PPOs also have catastrophic caps or limits, usually separate, but they seem to be significantly higher than the regional plan limitations.

1.6 Special Needs Plans (SNP)

Special Needs Plans (SNP) are Medicare Advantage coordinated care plans that target three specific groups of Medicare beneficiaries as special needs individuals:

- Institutionalized beneficiaries.

- Those who are dually entitled to Medicare and Medicaid.

- Other high-risk groups of chronically ill or disabled individuals who would benefit from enrollment in this type of plan.

These plans must offer Part D prescription drug benefits.

The first category of institutionalized beneficiaries includes those with an actual or anticipated stay of at least 90 days in a Skilled Nursing Facility, a nursing home, an inpatient psychiatric facility, or an intermediate care facility for the intellectually disabled. (Note that the government still uses the term "intermediate care facilities for the mentally retarded.") In some cases, these plans will accept as members those beneficiaries who qualify for institutional care, but who may live at home or some other place.

The second category of dual-eligible beneficiaries is specifically meant for those who have Medicare and full Medicaid benefits, and not meant for those who may be getting help with their Medicare premiums, deductibles, and coinsurance. While dual-eligibles should be cautious in joining a Medicare Advantage Plan, these SNPs are an exception, as they are specifically designed to get these two programs to work together for you.

You should know that SNPs have to make provisions with their providers, so that their providers either take the plan's payment as payment in full for any Part A and Part B services, or the provider bills the Medicaid program for any remainder (e.g., a co-payment). The SNP cannot ask the beneficiary for any payment. In fact, this protection applies to all dual-eligible beneficiaries in other types of plans as well.

The third category includes a number of different health conditions and diseases that can qualify a beneficiary to enroll in one of these SNPs. While this list is not exhaustive, and what is available differs widely from place to place, the following are conditions and diseases that could qualify you for an SNP:

- Asthma

- Cardiovascular disease

- Chronic obstructive pulmonary disease (COPD)

- Dementia
- Diabetes
- End-stage renal disease
- Human immunodeficiency virus (HIV)
- Hypertension

You need to be aware of one unique characteristic of these SNPs. If you are discharged from an institution, lose your Medicaid eligibility, or in the unusual case that your condition improves so much that you no longer meet the plan's disease criterion, you will have to disenroll from the plan. However, you will get a special enrollment period of three months in which you can join another Medicare Advantage Plan in your area if you wish. If you prefer, you can go into Original Medicare.

One new requirement is that SNPs must work with each beneficiary to develop an individual plan of care. This has to be based on an assessment of each beneficiary's unique needs; it must specify the goal or objective that the plan will strive to achieve for the beneficiary; and it must detail what services it will provide to meet the beneficiary's goal or objective.

One special service you may get with your SNP is a care coordinator. Sometimes this is a health professional, typically a nurse, who helps make sure you are taking your medicines, staying on the diet you were advised to follow, getting appointments to see the right physicians at the appropriate times, and monitoring your symptoms. You might also be assigned a social worker if you are a beneficiary dually-entitled to Medicare and Medicaid to make sure that you are using the plan's resources, and even the community resources you need, to manage your care situation. Much of this care coordination is done over the phone. Be aware that you will also need to follow your plan's rules on referrals and

prior authorizations, and you should get your coordinator to help you with this aspect of managed care.

It is important to note that an SNP can be any type of plan such as a Health Maintenance Organization or Private Fee-for-Service. You will need to follow your plan's general rules as well as any that deal with your specific condition or situation.

1.7 Private Fee-for-Service (PFFS) plans

Private Fee-for-Service (PFFS) plans are a fairly new type of Medicare Advantage Plan and they are basically a hybrid of fee-for-service and managed care. Members of a PFFS can go to any doctor, hospital, or provider in the US that is eligible to be paid by Medicare and is willing to accept the plan's terms of payment. However, if the PFFS plan has a network of providers (and most do not), your cost sharing will usually be higher if you get your care from a nonnetwork provider.

The PFFS plans work in a similar way to Original Medicare rather than managed care, because most of these plans do not have networks. You typically can go to any doctor, hospital, or provider who is approved by Medicare to be in the Medicare program, and who is willing to accept the payment terms of your plan. Most of the PFFS plans set the payment amount for a given service as the same as Original Medicare would pay. However, some doctors' offices are unfamiliar with PFFS plans, partly because the plans are new, or they are confused by the fact that there is a number of different PFFS plans operating in their locality, and so refuse, or are quite reluctant, to take beneficiaries who are enrolled in these PFFS plans.

Another thing you should be aware of is that it is legal for providers, including physicians and hospitals, to charge you more than the PFFS plan's payment terms. This is the amount the plan pays and whatever you have to pay (i.e., your coinsurance, co-payment, and/or deductible), which can be 15 percent or more, and you will be entirely responsible for paying. Very few plans permit this, but just to be safe double check with the PFFS plan about this before you enroll.

Many PFFS plans offer a Part D benefit. If you sign up with one that has the Part D prescription drug benefit, you have to use it. However, if the PFFS plan you sign up with does not offer this, you can join any stand-alone Part D plan and get your prescription drug coverage that way.

1.8 Medical Savings Accounts (MSA)

Medical Savings Accounts (MSAs) are very different from other Medicare Advantage Plans, and you should know that these plans are for the financially secure. Only a handful of Medicare beneficiaries choose this type of plan. MSA plans are premium-free.

If you join an MSA, you get an annual lump-sum deposit in a trust or custodial bank account in your name, which is your Medicare Advantage MSA. The bank is chosen by your plan. (You are allowed to change your bank.) These deposits are about $1,250 for a whole year. You will get a credit or debit card from the bank to use to pay your medical expenses; it will keep track of these expenses. Your bank may charge you custodial or maintenance fees, but it also may pay you interest, which is tax free. Your bank will send you a statement (Form 1099-SA) reporting your MSA distributions each January. You need this to file your federal income taxes. Interestingly, if you have money in your MSA at the time of your death, your spouse, if one survives you, can use this balance to pay for his or her own medical expenses.

Your plan also gives a high deductible medical insurance policy, which is similar to a catastrophic policy because it pays nothing until your out-of-pocket medical expenses hit a certain limit. Again, these limits vary, but will be approximately $3,000 a year. You will have to pay all your medical expenses until you reach your plan's deductible amount; it will pay all of your expenses after that. Medical expenses means only what Original Medicare would cover and the amount it would pay for it.

With few exceptions, health-care providers can charge you only the Medicare-approved amount for the service unless your physician does not take assignment, in which case the limiting charge applies at no more than 15 percent higher than the nonparticipating approved amount. Medicare here means what Part A and Part B, but not Part D, covers. Any covered Medicare Part A or Part B service you pay for — up to the amount Medicare would pay for it whether from your MSA or from your own wallet — counts toward meeting your deductible amount and it is not taxed.

It is your choice as to whether or not you use your MSA to pay for your medical bills. You are not required to do so, and some well-off beneficiaries take this route to accumulate tax-free funds. Note also that you can use your MSA to pay for any Qualified Medical Expenses and they are not taxed. A Qualified Medical Expense is any Medicare covered service, plus any service or item recognized by the Internal Revenue Service (IRS) as qualifying for a medical tax deduction. For example, if you get a hearing aid and pay for it using your MSA, that money is not taxed. The IRS list of what qualifies as medical expenses is much more extensive than Medicare's list. IRS Publication 502, "Medical and Dental Expenses," lists covered and noncovered expenses.

There are a number of restrictions on joining an MSA; for example, you can't join if you have health insurance that would cover any expenses that would count toward your deductible. Unlike other Medicare Advantage Plans, if you become covered by any such health insurance plan, you have to leave your MSA plan.

You cannot get Part D prescription drug coverage from an MSA plan, but you can join any stand-alone Part D plan in your area. Any money you pay for its premiums, deductibles, co-payments, and coinsurance does not count toward your MSA deductible (as these are not Part A or Part B items), but they are Qualified Medical Expenses that you can use your MSA money to pay for, if you wish.

1.9 Cost plans

According to Medicare officials, the Cost plans and the Demonstration plans (discussed next) are not technically Medicare Advantage Plans because they are authorized under different sections of the Medicare statute than the other Medicare Advantage Plans. However, from the beneficiary's point of view, they are simply different kinds of plans, and importantly, the same rights and protections apply to those who join these plans as the others. For simplicity, we'll refer to all Medicare managed care arrangements as Medicare Advantage Plans.

Cost plans are entities that are reimbursed by Medicare on a now old-fashioned payment method, and no new Cost plans are permitted to enter the Medicare program. If one exists where you live, you can still join. As these entities are survivors from an older era; they continue to have some rules that are generally no longer in effect, but which may be of interest to you. There are three unique rules about Cost plans:

- You do not have to have both Medicare Part A and Part B to join — you can also join if you have Part B only.

- You can join and leave the Cost plans in any month because there is no lock in.

- If you go outside your Cost plan's service area or network and get a Medicare-covered service, Medicare will pay its share of it as if you were in Original Medicare. (You will be responsible for any deductible, coinsurance, and excess charge amounts.)

Note that your Cost plan will be responsible for any emergency or urgently needed care you get, even if it's out-of-network.

You should definitely consider Cost plans if you do not have Part A. This is because as long as you go in-network, you can get the plan to pay for Part A services such as inpatient hospitalization. Be warned: If you don't have Part A and you get a Part A service outside your Cost plan's network, you have to pay the full cost as Part A of Original Medicare will not pay anything for it.

Some of the Cost plans offer a Part D benefit, while others don't. If the plan does not offer Medicare prescription drug coverage, you can join a stand-alone Medicare drug plan or stay in the one you are already in.

In general, Cost plans tend to have high monthly premiums. Also note that Cost plans do not provide extra or free additional benefits or savings on your Medicare Part B or Part D premiums like some other types of plans do.

1.10 Demonstration plans

From time to time Medicare will use its special legal authority to set up a special plan as a demonstration or pilot project. The idea is to try out new kinds of arrangements designed to improve care, particularly to a very targeted population or area, or to see if alternate reimbursement approaches would work, or to improve quality of care.

One such demonstration in 2009 concerned improving quality of services to end-stage renal disease beneficiaries. This Demonstration plan is available only in selected areas. Generally, beneficiaries with this disease cannot join a Medicare Advantage Plan, so people with end-stage renal disease may wish to look into this type of plan as it may help with medical costs and improve health by focusing on quality care.

1.11 PACE plans

In an effort to quell rising Medicaid costs of nursing home care, and to provide an alternative to them and a better quality of life, the PACE alternative to nursing homes was first established as the On-Loc program in San Francisco. This program tries to keep people out of nursing homes and in a residential setting (preferably their own home) by providing an array of medical and long-term care services, in the belief that these are superior both in terms of cost and quality compared to nursing home care. Many of the PACE programs' services are given in adult day care centers, and they arrange for transportation to these centers. Not all states have PACE plans, and even within states that do, only certain areas provide this plan option.

Most Medicare Advantage information correctly indicates that programs for all-inclusive care for the elderly or PACE plans are Medicaid managed care plans run by individual states' Medicaid programs, and that most beneficiaries in them are fully eligible for both Medicaid and Medicare. What is not usually explained clearly is that beneficiaries that have Medicare but not Medicaid may also join these plans. While these Medicare-only beneficiaries have to pay a steep monthly premium for long-term care (and also a Part D premium because they have to get their prescription drug coverage through the plan), this may be an attractive alternative to paying out-of-pocket for nursing home care or assistive

care in one's own home. This may be especially true because under PACE you don't pay deductibles or co-payments for either medical care or for drugs.

Note that even though these are technically Medicaid plans, you have the right, if you leave your PACE plan, to get a special enrollment period to join a Medicare Advantage Plan or to go into Original Medicare and get the right to purchase a Medigap policy.

2. Enrolling in or Disenrolling from a Medicare Advantage Plan

Let's first talk about when you can join a Medicare Advantage Plan or Part C. You should be aware that these rules have changed since Part D has gone into effect. This is because most Part C plans also offer Part D coverage, and there are restrictions on when you can sign up for Part D. Some of these restrictions have in turn been imposed on Part C so you can't circumvent the restrictions on getting Part D.

The Medicare program guarantees you certain times that you can sign up. The following sections will discuss the enrollment periods available to you.

2.1 Initial coverage election period

This enrollment period gives you the opportunity to join a Medicare Advantage Plan when you first get both Medicare Part A and Part B. While this is often when you turn age 65 or get Medicare because of your disability, it applies at other times too.

The vast majority of Medicare beneficiaries get Part A and Part B during their Part B initial enrollment period. This is the three months before, the month of, and the three months after you first become eligible for Medicare. Your opportunity to sign up for a Medicare Advantage

Plan is the same seven months as your opportunity to enroll in Part B.

When you get into your Medicare Advantage Plan it can be just a little tricky because it depends on when you enroll in Part B and sign up for your plan. For most people this will be quite simple, as they will automatically get their Part B the month they become 65 or are on disability for 25 months. If they also sign up for their plan in any of the three months before they get Part B, they will be enrolled in their plan the same month they get Part B.

If you don't sign up (or get automatically signed up) for Part B before you get your Medicare Part A, there is a delay of up to two months after you sign up until you actually get your Part B.

Not all Medicare beneficiaries want to enroll in Part B as soon as they become eligible. Usually, this is because they continue to work and are covered by an employer or union group health plan. You may recall that when they lose this coverage, usually because they retire, they get an opportunity to enroll in Part B without any penalty. Since this is their first enrollment in Part B, it's the first time they have Part A and Part B, and they get their Initial Coverage Election Period in conjunction with this. For these beneficiaries, this is the three months immediately preceding their entitlement to both Part A and Part B.

There are some rare situations in which the Initial Coverage Election Period may begin, such as for a beneficiary who has Part B, and then earns enough quarters of coverage to get Part A. Since this is the first time the beneficiary has both Part A and Part B, he or she gets a chance to enroll in Part C at this time.

2.2 General enrollment period

The general enrollment period is a special case of the Initial Coverage Election Period (ICEP) discussed in section **2.1**. You may recall from Chapter 1 that everyone who is eligible for Part B but does not have it may enroll in it during the Part B general enrollment period that lasts from January 1 to March 31 of every year. If you enroll during this time, you will get your Part B on July 1. If you already have Part A, as of that date, you will now have both Part A and B, and thus become eligible for Part C. You may sign up for a Medicare Advantage Plan in the three months preceding your entitlement to Part B; that is, you must enroll between April 1 and June 30. Your enrollment into your plan will be effective July 1, as that is when you get Part B. There is one hitch: You can't sign up for a Part C plan that includes Part D as you could have enrolled in Part D when you just had your Part A.

2.3 Open enrollment for newly eligible individuals

The open enrollment for newly eligible individuals exists for those beneficiaries who already had their initial election enrollment period, which they may or may not have used to join a Medicare Advantage Plan. If you enroll or re-enroll in Part B, you are now newly eligible to join a Medicare Advantage Plan because you now meet the requirements of having both Part A and Part B. This opportunity is rarely used, but it could indeed be a help to some beneficiaries.

You must sign up in the first three months you have both Part A and Part B, or before December 31 of that year, whichever is first. You will be enrolled the first of the month after the month you enroll in a plan. Note that you cannot change your Part D entitlement status so if you have Part D; you have to join a Medicare Advantage Plan that has Part D or you can join a plan that does not have Part D and just stay in your Part D plan. If you don't have Part D, you can join any plan that does not offer Part D coverage.

For example, suppose you began receiving your Medicare on August 1, 2009, and accepted your enrollment into Part B. You also joined a Part D stand-alone drug plan because you have to take some medications. Because these medications made you better, you dropped your Part B after three months, effective on November 1. You then had second thoughts, and signed up for it during the 2010 general enrollment period, and your Part B resumed on July 1, 2010. You now have both Part A and Part B, and you have a chance to enroll in a Medicare Advantage Plan during July, August, or September of 2010. If you do enroll, it will be effective the month after you sign up. You must keep your Part D entitlement by signing up for a Medicare Advantage Plan that has Part D coverage, or sign up for a plan that does not have Part D and so permits you to keep your current Part D stand-alone plan.

2.4 Annual election period

Almost every Medicare Advantage Plan is required to have open enrollment from November 15 to December 31 of every year so you can join. (You may also see the Annual Election Period or Open Enrollment referred to as the Annual Coordinated Election Period.) If you are in Original Medicare, you can sign up for a Medicare Advantage Plan during this time frame or, if you are in a plan, you can change from one plan to another. If you want to leave your plan, and go back to Original Medicare, you can do that as well. If you have Part D through your Medicare Advantage Plan, but leave it, you can join a stand-alone Part D plan. (You will note that this time window is identical to the annual Part D open enrollment period.) All these changes will be effective on January 1.

2.5 Open enrollment period

During each calendar year's open enrollment period, which lasts from January 1 through March 31, you can make changes with one major restriction: You cannot change your Part D entitlement status. That is, if you are not entitled to Part D, you can't get it. If you are in Part D, you have to stay in it. If you use the open enrollment period, the change takes effect the first of the month following the month you make the change (it will always be February 1, March 1, or April 1). Just so you know, a Medicare Advantage Plan does not have to accept new enrollments in this period, but most do.

If you are in a Medicare Advantage Plan, you can switch to another one or go into Original Medicare. If you are not in a Medicare Advantage Plan, you can sign up for one. If you have Part D and you are in a Medicare Advantage Plan, you can switch to another Medicare Advantage Plan as long as it has a Part D plan, too. You can also leave your Medicare Advantage Plan in which you also have Part D benefits, and go back to Original Medicare, but you have to simultaneously sign up for a stand-alone Part D plan.

If you are in Original Medicare and have a stand-alone Part D drug plan, you can join a Medicare Advantage Plan that has Part D, or one that doesn't and keep your current drug plan. If you don't have a Part D plan, you can only join a Medicare Advantage Plan with no drug coverage. If you are in a stand-alone Part D plan, you can't use this to change your Part D plan to another stand-alone plan because this is a Part C change period. Table 14 will help you understand this better.

A Medicare Advantage Plan does not have to take new members during this period. It can

TABLE 14

OPEN ENROLLMENT PERIOD DOS AND DON'TS

If your current coverage is the following:	You *can* use the open enrollment period to get the following:	You *cannot* use the open enrollment period to get the following:
Medicare Advantage with prescription drug coverage	A different Medicare Advantage Plan with prescription drug coverage **or** Original Medicare and a stand-alone prescription drug plan	A Medicare Advantage Plan with no prescription drug coverage **and** Original Medicare and no stand-alone prescription drug plan
Medicare Advantage with no prescription drug coverage	A different Medicare Advantage Plan with no prescription drug coverage **or** Original Medicare and no stand-alone prescription drug plan	Medicare Advantage with prescription drug coverage **and** Original Medicare and a stand-alone prescription drug plan
Original Medicare and a stand-alone prescription drug plan	A Medicare Advantage Plan with prescription drug coverage	A Medicare Advantage Plan with no prescription drug coverage **and** A different prescription drug plan to use with Original Medicare
Original Medicare and no stand-alone prescription drug plan	A Medicare Advantage Plan with no prescription drug coverage	Medicare Advantage with prescription drug coverage **And** Original Medicare and a stand-alone drug plan

accept new members during only a part of this time frame and not the whole three months. If you are thinking of switching plans, call the plan you are considering joining.

If you want to switch from a Medicare Advantage organization to Original Medicare, the way you use this option is you join a stand-alone prescription drug plan. This will also disenroll you from your Part C plan.

2.6 Special enrollment periods

Special enrollment periods are the occasions when you get a special opportunity to change your Medicare Advantage status. You can change your status by switching from one Medicare Advantage Plan to another, to go from Original Medicare into a plan, or to go from a plan back to Original Medicare. In this last case you are generally afforded the right to get a Medigap policy, which may be critical to you. Be aware that this right only applies during special enrollment periods.

You should know that special enrollment periods end when the time frame for that period ends, or when you elect a Medicare Advantage Plan. For example, you may be in a special enrollment period and you disenroll from a Medicare Advantage Plan, and then go into Original Medicare. You then have second thoughts, and you join a Medicare Advantage Plan. As long as you do this within the special enrollment period, that's fine; the intervening time in Original Medicare doesn't end the enrollment period, but enrolling in your new plan does.

2.6a Permanent change of residence

Perhaps the most important special enrollment period is when you permanently change your residence to a place outside the area your Medicare Advantage Plan serves. This period begins not necessarily when you move, but depends on when you tell your Medicare Advantage Plan that you did or will move. You have to prepare ahead of time to make sure that the health care you need is covered.

As part of your moving preparations, find out if your current Medicare Advantage Plan does or does not include your new place of residence. If it does not, you need to use your new zip code and go to the Medicare website to find out what is available. When you move, you can contact the new plan you want to join and enroll. Or, if you decide you don't want to join a Medicare Advantage Plan, you have the right to get a Medigap policy if you want one. (See Chapter 10 for details.)

You should be aware of something here. If you contact your old plan and tell them you are moving, they have to begin disenrolling you. That is, this will establish the time frame for your special enrollment period. It might be better to wait until you have a new plan that you are ready to enroll with and when you do, it will automatically disenroll you from your old plan effective the date you join your new plan. This way you will be continuously covered. You can do this any time in the six months after your move, but *do not miss that deadline*. If you miss the deadline, you will lose your special enrollment period and, since you can't join a plan, you will automatically be put into Original Medicare.

You really need to find a plan you want to join before you move. One reason you may wait until you move to join a new plan is that you may be going to an area where you are clueless about the medical community, and want to take some time to research it. Remember that if you get medical care in your new area before you join a new plan, you will always have the hassle of dealing with out-of-area services. Another reason to wait is that you may have scheduled a service with your old plan (e.g., surgery), and you really want to have the surgeon you picked to do it. In cases such as these, you want to be careful about when you change plans.

If you notify your Medicare Advantage Plan of your intended move no later than the month before you actually move, your special enrollment period will begin with the month immediately before the month you actually move, and will continue for three more months (the month you move and the two months thereafter). For example, you are planning to move on July 10. You notify your plan on May 20. Your special enrollment period begins June 1, and goes to September 30.

If you notify your Medicare plan in the month you actually move, or in the six months after that, your special enrollment period begins in the month you notify your plan, and goes on for two more months, for a total of three months. For example, suppose you move on September 5. You notify your plan later that month, on September 20. Your special enrollment period begins September 1 and goes through November 30.

Your change can be effective no earlier than the month you actually move, and no earlier than the month you give notification, but it can be effective for up to three months after the month you give notification; that is, you get to choose in which of these months it becomes effective.

2.6b Employer and union group health plan changes

A special enrollment period exists for beneficiaries to help coordinate employer and union group health plans and Medicare Advantage options. These apply to beneficiaries who are —

- enrolling into or out of an employer or union sponsored Medicare Advantage Plan,
- disenrolling from a Medicare Advantage Plan to enroll in an employer or union group health plan, and
- disenrolling from an employer or union group health plan to enroll in a Medicare Advantage Plan.

For example, suppose you are a Medicare beneficiary who is still working and covered by an employer or union group health plan. You retire and you are no longer covered by that health plan. You get a special enrollment period to sign up for a Medicare Advantage Plan. If you were covered by such a group health plan, you might not have had Part B. You will now also get the option to join Part B and, once you have it, to enroll in a Medicare Advantage Plan.

This special enrollment period is available to individuals who have an employer or union group health plan and it ends two months after the month the employer or union coverage ends. You may choose an effective date of up to three months after the month in which you complete

an enrollment request to join a Medicare Advantage Plan. However, the effective date may not be earlier than the first of the month following the month in which the request was made.

Another example is that you retired and after a while you go back to work. After you are at the new job for a certain period, you earn the chance to join your employer group health plan. You decide you want to join the Medicare Advantage Plan. You can do so if you join in the time frame that your employer group health plan allows, even though you may not be in a period when you can ordinarily join or change a Medicare Advantage Plan.

You can also join a plan when the employer or union group health plan allows you to make changes in your health coverage choices, such as during the employer's or union's open season, or at other times the employer or union allows. Sometimes these open seasons do not coincide with the usual times you can join Medicare Advantage Plans. The special enrollment period allows changes in the time frames specified by the employer or union group health plan.

2.6c Extra help or low-income subsidy Part D Medicare beneficiaries

If you qualify for Part D extra help or low-income subsidy, you have a special enrollment period that begins the month you become eligible for this subsidy and continues every month as long as you are eligible for it.

This special enrollment period allows you to disenroll from and enroll in a different Part D drug plan or a Medicare Advantage Plan with Part D coverage at any time. Your change is effective with the first of the month immediately following your election. The special enrollment period allows you to change enrollment on a monthly basis. This includes any change as long as you keep Part D drug coverage, and so it includes going from one Part D stand-alone plan to another, or from one Medicare Advantage Plan with Part D to another, or from a Part D stand-alone plan to a Medicare Advantage Plan with Part D, or vice versa. Note that while Medicare guidance isn't clear, this does not allow you to change your Medicare Advantage Plan that does not have Part D to another such plan.

It is possible because of a change in your financial or family arrangements that you lose your low-income subsidy or extra help. Typically, you will get a notice of this late in the calendar year. If you lose your low-income subsidy, you will have a special enrollment period to make a change during the three-month period of January through March of the next year. This allows you to keep your current drug plan through to the end of the year, and then change it in the beginning of the next year.

Sometimes beneficiaries lose their eligibility for the low-income subsidy during the year; this is due to a change in marital status. The loss of the subsidy is typically effective in the month after the event is reported to the Social Security Administration. This special enrollment period begins the month you are notified of the loss and continues for two months. This gives these beneficiaries the opportunity to look for a drug plan that perhaps has a lower premium or better benefit structure than the one they had.

The effective date for all enrollments under this low-income subsidy special enrollment period is the first day of the month following the drug plan's receipt of the enrollment request. For example, suppose you are awarded a low-income subsidy, and the Centers for Medicare & Medicaid Services automatically enrolls you into a Part D drug plan effective October 1. In November, you decide you would rather be enrolled in another Part D drug plan or a Medicare Advantage Plan with the Part D drug

benefit and you submit a request. You do so using the special enrollment period; your enrollment is effective December 1.

2.6d Medicare or Medicaid enrollment and disenrollment

If you have Medicare and Medicaid, you can join or leave a Medicare Advantage Plan at any time. Your request will be effective on the first of the very next month after you make the request. This includes beneficiaries who have full Medicaid entitlement (i.e., dual-eligibles) and those who receive help or cost sharing assistance from Medicaid, sometimes called partial dual-eligibles.

If your Medicaid entitlement or assistance ends, you can join or leave a Medicare Advantage Plan that month or in the following two months.

2.6e Open Enrollment Period for Institutionalized Individuals

If you move into or out of certain health-care facilities (e.g., nursing home or rehab hospital), you get a continuous Open Enrollment Period for Institutionalized Individuals. If you are admitted into a health care facility for an actual or anticipated length of stay (i.e., 90 days or longer), you can enroll into or disenroll from a Medicare Advantage Plan, or change plans at any time. Your request will be effective on the first of the very next month after you make it.

If you leave such an institution, you can join or leave a plan the month you leave the facility or the following two months. Note that those in Medicare Advantage Special Needs Plans qualify for this special enrollment period.

2.6f Loss of credible drug coverage

Because loss of credible drug coverage was discussed in detail in Chapter 6, section 2.3b, this section will be kept brief. If you have insurance that has creditable drug coverage, and you lose this insurance, or your creditable drug coverage is reduced so it is no longer creditable, you get a special enrollment period to join a Part D drug plan or a Medicare Advantage Plan with a Part D prescription drug benefit. You can join any Part D stand-alone plan in your area, but only a Medicare Advantage Plan with a Part D drug benefit. In other words, this special enrollment period has to be used to replace your loss of creditable drug coverage.

The special enrollment period begins with the month in which you are advised or notified of the loss or reduction of your creditable coverage. It ends two months after either the loss or reduction occurs or you receive this notice, whichever is later. If you do use this special enrollment period to join a Part D drug plan or a Medicare Advantage Plan with a Part D plan, the effective date of your new coverage may be the first of the month after the date you enroll.

2.6g You were never notified of non-creditable drug coverage

If you were never notified of non-creditable drug coverage, you can get a special enrollment period only with the written approval of the Centers for Medicare & Medicaid Services.

If you never received a notice that your health insurance drug coverage was not creditable, or if you never got a notice that your coverage went from creditable to non-creditable, you can get a special enrollment period to join either a Part D stand-alone plan or a Medicare Advantage Plan with drug coverage.

2.6h Nonrenewals

If your Medicare Advantage Plan decides it wants to leave Medicare, or if it reduces its service area so you are no longer in it, you will be given the opportunity to join another plan, and you will receive a notice from your plan explaining the details. These changes almost always

occur on January 1, and you will hear about it the previous October, so you have time to find another plan.

One very important thing to be aware of is that once your plan has actually left, Medicare will automatically put you into Original Medicare if you have not already joined another plan.

2.6i Terminations, sanctions, and contract violations

If the government decides to remove a plan from the Medicare Advantage program, it terminates its contract with that plan, and you will get a notice about what is happening, and what your options are. If this happens to you, you may be automatically enrolled in a similar plan, but also given the opportunity to change to another plan or return to Original Medicare. You will also be given the right to get a Medigap policy if you decide on Original Medicare.

The Centers for Medicare & Medicaid Services has the authority to sanction a Medicare Advantage Plan if it violated its contract with Medicare. This is a lesser-level punishment than a government-demanded contract termination. If your plan is sanctioned, and you were adversely affected by the action that gave rise to the sanction (e.g., inappropriate or illegal marketing to Medicare beneficiaries), you can ask for a special enrollment period to leave it or to join another plan.

The Centers for Medicare & Medicaid Services has the authority to decide if you were mistreated by your Medicare Advantage Plan by its action or inaction. For example, suppose it made misrepresentations to you when you joined the plan. If this is your situation, contact your Centers for Medicare & Medicaid Services regional office, or your State Health Insurance Assistance Program (SHIP). If the government finds in your favor, you will be given this special enrollment period that you can use to either go into Original Medicare (with the right to buy a Medigap policy) or to join another Medicare Advantage Plan.

2.6j Loss of Medicaid eligibility while in a Special Needs Plan

If you are a dual-eligible beneficiary, and lose your Medicaid eligibility while in a Medicare Advantage Special Needs Plan, there is some leeway for when your plan must disenroll you when you no longer qualify. Your Special Needs Plan must give you at least 30 days' notice before it disenrolls you and, at its option, can keep you for up to six months before it disenrolls you. When you are disenrolled, you will have a special enrollment period as determined by the Centers for Medicare & Medicaid Services for your involuntary disenrollment. Typically, this period is the month of disenrollment and the following two months.

If you are enrolled in a Medicare Advantage Special Needs Plan because of a particular condition, and your condition is cured or healed, you will have to disenroll. You will get a special enrollment period of three months in which you can join another Medicare Advantage Plan in your area if you wish.

2.6k Members of a qualified State Pharmacy Assistance Program

If you are newly enrolled in a qualified State Pharmacy Assistance Program, you have the right to a special enrollment period. Contact your program to discuss this.

3. End-Stage Renal Disease and Medicare Advantage

If you have end-stage renal disease, you generally cannot join a Medicare Advantage Plan; however, there are some exceptions. If you have end-stage renal disease and have a successful kidney transplant, you can, if you document your condition, join a Medicare Advantage Plan. If you are in a managed care plan and you get end-stage renal disease, and then you get Medicare, you can, if your current managed care plan is also a Medicare Advantage Plan, enroll in that plan as a Medicare beneficiary. (Sometimes this is called converting.)

If you prospectively enroll in a Medicare Advantage Plan and get end-stage renal disease in the months before your enrollment is effective, your enrollment remains valid.

If you are a Medicare beneficiary in a Medicare Advantage Plan and get end-stage renal disease, you can always continue your enrollment. However, you are not allowed to change from one plan to another, and if you leave your Medicare Advantage Plan and go back to Original Medicare, you can't rejoin any plan.

There is an exception and that is if your Medicare Advantage organization has a different Medicare Advantage Plan in the state you live in, and you move into that plan's service area, you can join that plan. Note that this means the same organization in the same state.

Another exception is if you are unlucky enough to be in a plan that terminates its Medicare contract (whether at its own request or because Medicare does so), you have one opportunity to join another Medical Advantage Plan. In this case, you can use the special enrollment period to join another plan.

A final exception is if you have employer or union health coverage, and as part of this you can enroll in a Medicare Advantage Plan, that plan can make exceptions to the "No End-Stage Renal Disease Beneficiaries" rule in a variety of circumstances. These exceptions are not on a case-by-case basis; they have to apply to everyone, and the plan can decide each calendar year whether or not to make exceptions. Consult with your employer or group health benefits administrator if you have this coverage and end-stage renal disease.

4. The Grandfather Clause

This section won't apply to anyone new to Medicare, but only to some of you who have been in it for quite some time. It is possible, even if you have only Part B and not Part A, that if you were in a Medicare Advantage Plan on December 31, 1998, and you are still in it, that you are getting Part A benefits from your plan. You may be paying a supplemental premium to your plan for these benefits. If you are one of these beneficiaries, you are grandfathered in because you can no longer join a Medicare Advantage Plan unless you have both Part A and Part B. If you are in this situation, and you don't pay the premium, you may be completely disenrolled. If you disenroll from your Medicare Advantage Plan or join another such organization, you will no longer meet the requirements for grandfathering, and will have to get Part A to join another Medicare Advantage Plan.

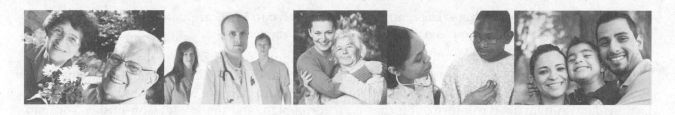

9
Part C: Researching and Managing
Medicare Advantage Plans

Finding the right Medicare Advantage Plan for you is best done by considering both cost and quality. You'll get a good idea of what a plan will cost you by comparing differing plans and what their benefit structures are by looking through the Medicare website. You should also consider the quality and reputation of the plan by using the Medicare website information and by consulting some other sources, such as on the Internet or at your local library.

You should make sure that any plan combining Part C and Part D gets you the medicines you need and is the best financial deal.

You may wish to use the Medicare Advantage Decision Sheets to help you compare the plans available to you. These sheets are included on the CD under the names "Drug and Quality Comparisons" and "Cost Comparisons."

1. Researching Plans

Besides looking at the Medicare and the Centers for Medicare & Medicaid Services websites for information on whether a plan is a good one to join or not, there are other sources you can look at as well.

You might also want to check out *US News & World Report's* ranking of health plans, which they have done for several years in a row. The plan rankings appear in the magazine in the fall. This ranking includes a section on Medicare plans that will help you figure out what plans are well-known and respected.

You may also wish to read *Consumer Reports* magazine, which has surveyed its readership about their managed care experiences for some time. You may be able to get some ideas, from a consumer's point of view, of a plan you are in or thinking of joining.

Another approach you may wish to take is looking at the accreditation information of the organization you are considering joining. While the Medicare program recognizes a number of organizations that accredit managed care outfits, only one of these, the National Committee for Quality Assurance (NCQA), works exclusively in this field. Unfortunately, few managed care organizations apply to this body for accreditation.

Another accreditation organization also has information available on its website. It's the Utilization Review Accreditation Commission

(URAC), which reviews a very large array of health care organizations. You can access the accreditation directory on its website.

A number of state governments make available reports on health care quality and satisfaction data, similar to the information that is beginning to appear on the Medicare website. At this point in time, only a few states are compiling this data and making it available to consumers. On some of their websites you can get bonus information on the performance of other health-care providers, especially hospitals, which may be of interest to you. Some of the states that include this information on their websites are listed in the Resources file included on the CD.

Some state governments also include consumer complaint information, which is generally collected by the various state insurance commissioners' offices as they deal in complaints on all types of insurance entities, including managed care companies. This data ranges from the ratio of complaints compared to the size of the company to those with breakouts by policy service, claims, and marketing issues. The general rule of thumb is to avoid those managed care outfits with high ratios of complaints. The easiest way to access this information is to go to the National Association of Insurance Commissioners website (www.naic.org).

2. Common Marketing Scams

You should always be aware that plans have a huge incentive to get you to join. This section will discuss some of the specific scams, abuses, and frauds you may encounter from salespeople. Beware!

Be careful of those people who try to pressure you to join a plan. If someone tells you, "If you don't sign up by the end of this week, you will lose your Medicare," you will know that it isn't the right plan for you. After reading this book, you will know the system well enough to know your Medicare enrollment and disenrollment rights.

Another trick some salespeople pull is the "bait and switch." This technique happens when you inquire about a Medigap policy or a Part D drug plan, and the salesperson pushes you into signing up for his or her company's Medicare Advantage Plan. Again, do not let anyone pressure you.

You will also need to be on the lookout for deceitful representation. There have been situations in which salespersons have posed as Federal Medicare officials, sometimes showing red, white, and blue cards that look just like real Medicare cards. As Medicare officials will not come to your home, you should always call your local law enforcement if someone is posing as one.

Some agents deliberately lie about a plan's benefit structures or a beneficiary's potential liabilities to make their plan seem better than it really is. Some agents claim beneficiaries would not pay anything for medical care and would be penalized by Medicare if they do not sign up. Not wanting this penalty, beneficiaries, who are often dual-eligible, enroll in the plan. Dual-eligible beneficiaries who usually are better off in Original Medicare are particularly hurt with this type of marketing. This is why it is so important for you to research the plans you are interested in and understand the plan you are currently in to avoid situations like this one.

Another problem is aggressive telephone marketing. In this situation, sales agents make repeated phone calls to beneficiaries, which often become increasingly threatening, using scare tactics and misrepresentations. Beneficiaries have even been told that Medicare needs to send an agent to their homes to correct a mistake in the *Medicare & You* handbook that all beneficiaries receive. Contact your local law enforcement if this happens.

Watch out for fraudulent sign-ups. In this situation, sales representatives ask Medicare beneficiaries to complete a "request for more information form" or a form for a "free gift." However, what the beneficiaries actually sign is an enrollment form to join a plan. The beneficiaries never realize that they are in a new plan until a claim for service is denied by their Medicare Administrative Contractor.

Some salespeople gain access to an apartment, condo, or seniors' complex and go from door to door, seeking new signees to their plan. Once they secure one beneficiary, they ask the beneficiary to introduce him or her to friends and neighbors to sell his or her plan. Note that Medicare prohibits all unsolicited door-to-door calls.

There have also been some cases in which agents have told seniors that Medicare is going private. This is a scare tactic to get beneficiaries to join their plans. Don't sign up for a plan if you are unsure of what an agent is telling you.

Of course, these are not all the ways that beneficiaries are taken advantage of and none of these scams are new. With the proliferation of Medicare Advantage Plans, and the substantial sums that these companies receive from the government for each enrolled beneficiary, the sales activity has become very competitive.

2.1 Marketing restrictions on Medicare Advantage Plans

Medicare has a lot of rules and restrictions on methods you can be sold or marketed a Medicare Advantage Plan. These restrictions are placed on organizations in an effort to make sure you get good information and are not discriminated against. When dealing with plan representatives, keep the following Medicare marketing restrictions in mind:

- A salesperson may *not* come to your home uninvited.

- You cannot be charged a fee to enroll in a plan.

- A plan may not offer you any cash payment as an incentive to join its plan. The providers are allowed to give you gifts of a nominal value to attend a sales pitch, but can't give you meals or costly gifts.

- A plan may not send you unwanted emails.

- A plan may not cold call you.

- A plan may not enroll you in its plan over the telephone unless you have called them.

- A plan may never ask you for a payment by use of the telephone, the Internet, email, or in person. The plan has to send you a bill.

- A plan may not tell you that its plan is a "Medicare Supplement."

- A plan may not conduct sales activities at educational events (i.e., health fairs and community events) or in health-care providers' waiting rooms or at pharmacy counters.

- A plan must abide by state laws governing the licensing of agents and brokers, and federal law regarding training and testing.

- An agent, in meeting with you to sell you his or her plan, can only discuss the topics or products that you agreed to when making the appointment.

In enrolling you or reviewing your application, your plan cannot discriminate against you, especially if you may have a condition or one or more diseases that are very expensive to treat. The exceptions to this rule are that the plan must use information about end-stage renal disease and, if it is a Special Needs Plan enrolling beneficiaries with specific conditions, it must use information about those conditions. Generally, a plan may never use information concerning the following:

- Your medical condition, either physical or mental

- Your past medical claims experience

- Health care you may have received in the past

- Your prior receipt of health care

- Your medical history

- Genetic information about you

- Your disability

Plans have less of an incentive to discriminate medically than they used to because the payment methodology Medicare uses to pay plans now includes adjusting the payments for medical experience. However, you should nonetheless be aware of these special nondiscrimination provisions, particularly if you have a very expensive or difficult to treat condition.

The purpose of detailing all this is not to make you an expert on Medicare rules about marketing plans; in fact, there are even more rules than listed here. The purpose is to let you know what plans (and their representatives) can't do, so if you think the plan you are considering is doing something wrong, you are aware and can find another plan with better sales representatives. You should call your state insurance commissioner (the numbers are included in the Resources file on the CD) to complain. You might also want to call Medicare and file a complaint.

In addition to following the above rules, Private Fee-for-Service Plans must —

- make it clear that to you there is no guarantee that your doctor or hospital will agree to accept the plan's terms and conditions and provide you with treatment if you enroll in the plan;

- call you after you enroll to make sure that you wanted to join and that you understand how the plan works. If they are unable to reach you by phone, they must send you a letter with instructions on how to disenroll if you decide not to join;

- have people available to answer any questions you have about the plan and how it works; and

- have people available to answer your physician's or provider's questions about how the plan would work with him or her.

Medicare posts special information on its website that can help you decide if a plan is consumer-friendly. Specifically, it assigns ratings to indicate how well each plan is scored on consumer service. The Centers for Medicare & Medicaid Services provides on its website the names of plans that have been made to take corrective action, which is a very serious step for the government to take against plans that are not following the rules.

3. Important Plan Communications

You need to know about some of the communications that you will receive from your plan. Soon after joining it, you will get an identification card that you should always show when you have a health encounter. In these situations, don't use your red, white, and blue Medicare card — keep it in a safe place.

3.1 "Evidence of Coverage" booklet

You will receive an "Evidence of Coverage" booklet. This booklet will detail your health coverage and it contains specific information you need to know about exactly how the plan covers your care. It will also discuss what health services the plan will pay for, how much it will pay for them, and what cost sharing you will be responsible for. The more familiar you are with it, the better off you will be.

Your plan must describe its rules for how you access care while you are a member of the plan. This explanation must include rules on how to get primary care, hospital care, and other medical services. It has to clearly tell you how you get referrals for specialty care.

It will tell you if you have to choose a primary care physician to coordinate your care. If you do have to choose a physician, it will tell you how to do so, and it will also tell you how you can change your primary care physician.

As part of this service, it has to remind you to use its network of physicians, hospitals, and providers that are affiliated with the plan for all health-care services, except emergencies, urgently needed care, or out-of-area renal dialysis. Further, it has to explain its prior authorization rules for any in-network or out-of-network services and describe other review requirements that must be met in order to ensure payment for the services. The booklet must reiterate that the plan won't pay for out-of-network or unauthorized services if its rules are not met.

If your plan allows the use of non-plan or non-preferred providers, or has a "Point-of-Service" option, it has to explain this to you, and tell you if this will cost you more (it usually does), and by how much.

It must define what an "emergency medical condition" is and describe its rules for emergency care and for the coverage of post-stabilization care. The plan must explain that members are not required to go to plan-affiliated hospitals and practitioners when they experience an emergency. (If your plan covers emergencies outside the US, it has to discuss this, too.)

The booklet must define "urgent care" and explain that urgently needed care provided by non-plan providers is covered when a member is out of its service area, and describe its payment rules for urgent care.

It must tell you of your right to file a grievance, to request an initial determination, and to file an appeal. Furthermore, it must describe the mechanics of the processes involved in these situations. It must explain that you have the right to appeal any decision the organization or plan makes regarding a denial, termination, or reduction of services or benefits. This includes your right to appeal a denial of payment for a service after it has been given (post-service) as well as the denial of service prior to the service being given (pre-service).

3.2 Annual Notice of Change

Every year you will receive an Annual Notice of Change from your plan. You should receive the notice by October 31; if you don't, call your plan and ask to have one sent to you.

This document highlights the significant changes that the plan will be making effective January 1 of the next year. These changes can include additions or subtractions to the plan's provider networks; expanding or contracting the area it serves; raising or lowering its premiums; and changing its benefit structure, including co-payments, deductibles, and need for authorizations. If you have your Part D prescription drug coverage with your plan, the notice may list changes in formularies and tiers. Changes in the supplemental benefits will be included as well. You need to go through the notice carefully to decide if you want to stay with your plan or change.

This is a good time to contact your physicians and other important health-care providers to see if they are going to stay with your plan.

Their contracts usually go by calendar year, so most changes occur on January 1.

3.3 Physician or health provider leaves the plan

Your Medicare Advantage organization is required to communicate to you if a contracted physician or provider leaves a plan, if you have been seeing that physician or going to that provider on a regular basis. Your plan has to let you know in writing that this physician or health provider is leaving the network at least 30 calendar days in advance. In addition, if your primary care physician leaves your plan, your plan must notify you 30 days in advance in writing of this, even if you have not been going to this doctor on a regular basis, that is, must always notify you if your primary care physician leaves your plan. The notice in both instances will tell you how to make new arrangements. The distinction is that the plan must always notify the beneficiary when the primary physician leaves — even if the beneficiary has not been going to them. And, if a beneficiary has been reguarly seeing any other physician, they must notify the beneficiary when that physician leaves.

4. Special Care Situations

You should take time to become familiar with the special care situations discussed in the following sections because each of them is particular to Medicare Advantage care.

4.1 Emergency and urgently needed care

One of the most serious areas of disagreement between Medicare Advantage Plans and their beneficiary members are the issues of emergency care and urgently needed care. Both of these entail getting services provided outside the normal paths of approval and pre-authorization and/or using out-of-network health care. Plans always seem primed to question these occurrences, and to deny claims resulting from use of these services.

4.1a Medical emergency

A medical emergency is when you reasonably believe that your health is in serious danger — when every second counts. A medical emergency includes severe pain, a bad injury, a serious illness, or a medical condition that is rapidly getting much worse.

A more technical definition has some particular phrases that you should be aware of. This is included here to give you a better feel for just what emergency services are, but also to include some language you can use to appeal any dispute you may have with your plan in case it refuses to pay for what you believe it should. Specifically, Medicare defines a medical emergency as a condition comprised of symptoms of sufficient severity (including severe pain) such that a prudent layperson with an average knowledge of health and medicine could reasonably expect the absence of immediate medical care to result in serious jeopardy to the health of the individual, serious impairment to bodily functions, or serious dysfunction of any bodily organ or part.

This definition applies no matter what the final medical diagnosis turns out to be. To some degree, this is a subjective call. This can be to your advantage. The services provided include treating the condition, evaluating it, and stabilizing it.

You may face an issue of when this medical emergency rule stops applying and the rules for the normal authorization of services begin to apply. This is sometimes referred to as post-stabilization care. Your treating physician makes the decision as to when the emergency has ended and the regular care begins, and your Medicare Advantage Plan has to go along with him or her. That is, you can't be transferred to the care of the plan or its physicians, or discharged, unless your treating physician approves it. This will typically happen because your plan has to be contacted so it can arrange for your care, and your plan will take over your care, by putting its own physician in charge of your care or by coming to an agreement with your treating physician about what to do.

Once the treating physician says that your condition is not a medical emergency, any additional care you get must follow the usual rules your plan has, which typically means that you must get the care from a plan provider or have it pre-approved. The exception is that if you are not in your plan's service area, and the additional care you should get, while not care for a medical emergency, adheres to the definition of "urgently needed care," then your plan is still fully responsible.

You should know that no Medicare Advantage Plan can charge you more than $50 for emergency department services. This is to prevent plans from getting around your right to access emergency services by charging a high co-payment or coinsurance rate for this. Some plans charge less than this, and some will not even charge you if you are admitted to the hospital in the event of an emergency. A plan cannot charge you more for post-stabilization care than it would if you had received these services through your plan.

4.1b Urgent care

Urgently needed services are almost always defined as services you receive when you are away from your plan's area. These medical services must be —

- medically necessary and immediately required;

- the result of an unforeseen illness, injury, or condition; and

- given the circumstances, unreasonable for you to obtain through your plan's participating provider network.

For example, a plan enrollee has been under the care of an internist for years for a chronic stomach condition. However, while he was visiting his daughter, well out of his plan's service area, his condition flared up, causing considerable discomfort and an inability to eat normally. The beneficiary saw a local doctor who treated him and also changed his prescription dosage.

Even though the enrollee was well aware of the chronic condition, his flare-up was unforeseen. Although the flare-up was not a medical emergency, it did require immediate medical attention and it was unreasonable for the enrollee to return to the service area for treatment.

When medical services are urgently needed, that is, they meet the Medicare definition, your plan is obligated to take responsibility for the services. If the services meet the definition, just like emergency services, you do not require your plan's prior authorization.

Note that under very unusual circumstances, medical services may be considered urgently needed when you are in your plan's service area, but for some reason its provider network is temporarily unavailable or inaccessible. For example, suppose there is a bad storm in your area and you fall in your blacked-out home. You are hurt but you believe that you don't have a true emergency condition; however, you do need medical help as your pain is getting worse. You phone your plan for direction, but their phone system is down due to the storm. A neighbor drives you to the nearest emergency room. This would count as urgently needed care even though you are in the plan's area.

4.2 Direct access to care situations

There are times that you get services from your plan without getting a referral or pre-authorization, and one situation when you can always get out-of-area services:

- If you are a woman, you may, without referral, go to any in-network or plan provider or physician for your covered routine and preventive health care services. These include screening mammograms, Pap tests, and pelvic and breast exams. Be sure to observe any frequency limits followed by your plan. (These limits can't be more restrictive than those of Original Medicare.)

- You have the right to get a flu vaccine without referral. No plan can impose any cost sharing on flu or pneumonia vaccines. Just be sure to use an in-network provider if this is required of you.

- While this would apply to only a few beneficiaries, if you are traveling out-of-network and need kidney dialysis, you don't have to get plan approval or pre-authorization for this service. However, you should make sure the dialysis center you go to gets the payment arrangements worked out with your plan first.

4.3 Hospice care and Medicare Advantage

If you are in a Medicare Advantage Plan, you can elect the Medicare hospice benefit. Be aware that hospice benefits are always given outside of a Medicare Advantage Plan, directly by the hospice itself, or by caregivers it arranges for. When you elect this approach to care, your Medicare Advantage Plan can't treat you for your terminal illness.

If you are in Medicare hospice care, you can join a Medicare Advantage Plan; there is the inevitable exception, however, that if you are in hospice care, you cannot join a Medical Saving Account (MSA) plan. However, at this point there is probably very little reason to join a Medicare Advantage Plan unless it has some extra or special benefit, such as it pays your Part B premium or has a transportation benefit you need.

5. Your Special Rights and Protections in a Medicare Advantage Plan

As a Medicare beneficiary, you should know about the special and powerful rights and protections you have when you are in a Medicare Advantage Plan. The important thing that you must understand is that when you become a Medicare Advantage member, you are still entitled to receive all medically necessary services covered under Part A and Part B, and you also have special rights to use as an individual beneficiary to balance the power your Medicare Advantage Plan has over your care.

5.1 Change primary care physician

You have the right to choose and to change your primary care physician without interference. For example, you are assigned to a primary care physician you do not know, and it may be that you're not impressed with his or her skills. You can call your plan and get a change.

5.2 Choose health-care providers

You have the right to choose the health-care provider you want to use. That is, you have a voice in which physicians and providers you use and the right to choose them. However, you are usually restricted to providers within the plan's network.

5.3 Noninterference

One interesting protection you have is that Medicare Advantage Plans cannot restrict or prohibit any health professional, such as your doctor or a specialist you consult with, from advising you about your health status, or what appropriate medical care or treatment options exist for you. This includes the freedom to give you sufficient information so that you can decide what treatment options are best for you, and the risks, benefits, and consequences of treatment and nontreatment. Your plan cannot prohibit these health professionals advocating for you.

This noninterference provision exists because at times in managed care, a plan's internal rules on treatments and attempts to constrain costs may encourage caregivers toward one approach rather than another. While this protection does not change that, it does allow physicians and health professionals, even when part of the plan's structure, to tell you what they think you need to know.

5.4 Compensation arrangements

If you do feel that your treatment options suggested by your physician are being limited by cost constraints, you have the right to ask your plan about how these arrangements work. Medicare's literature has stated that "Medicare doesn't allow plans to pay doctors in a way that wouldn't let you get the care you need." This statement does not mean that plans, which get a fixed amount of money to cover its services, can't make incentive arrangements with caregivers that help them to control budgets. You have a right to know how your physician is compensated.

5.5 Second opinion

Just as in Original Medicare, you have the right to get a second opinion. Some plans will only help pay for a second opinion if you first get a referral from your primary care doctor. After you get a referral, you must get the second opinion from the doctor named in the referral. If you want to get a second opinion from a doctor who doesn't belong to your plan, talk to your plan first. In some cases, plans will help pay for a second opinion from a doctor outside the plan's network. If your plan won't pay, you could still get the second opinion from the doctor who doesn't belong to your plan, but you would have to pay the full cost.

If you are in a Medicare Advantage Preferred Provider Organization (PPO) or a Private Fee-for-Service Plan (PFFS), your plan will help pay for a second opinion. You probably don't need a referral. If you are in a PPO, you may have to pay more if you get a second opinion from a doctor who doesn't belong to your plan.

5.6 Cultural competence

You have the right to get care and services in a culturally competent way. This means that services have to be accessible to all beneficiaries, including those with language barriers, lack of literacy, or handicaps such as hearing difficulties. This includes getting care in a language you can understand and in a culturally sensitive manner.

5.7 Treatment plan

If you have a complex or serious medical condition, you have the right to get a treatment plan from your doctor. The purpose of this plan is that it lets you see a specialist within your Medicare Advantage Plan without a specific referral as many times as you and your doctor think you need, that is, whatever is in your individual plan.

5.8 Advance directives

When you first enroll, your plan has to give you written information on your rights under state law to make decisions concerning your medical care, including the right to accept or refuse treatment, and the right to formulate advance directives. It cannot discriminate against you because you have, or have not, executed an advance directive. It must annotate your medical record as to whether or not you have an advance directive. If your state law changes regarding these, it has to give you notice of this change.

Note: Advance directives include living wills and durable powers of attorney.

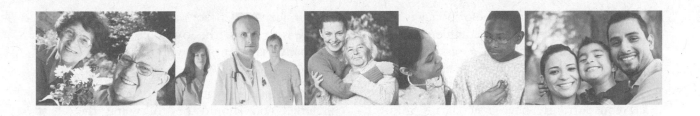

10
Medigap: Medicare Supplement Insurance

Medigap policies are private health insurance policies that many Medicare beneficiaries buy to help pay for the "gaps" in what Medicare does not pay for. (Note that Medigap is also known as Medicare Supplement Insurance.) Medigap policies are specifically engineered to work with and complement Medicare, so that you won't be paying for any overlapping coverage.

Medigap policies are well regulated by both federal and state law, and you have some very significant and protective rights under these laws, which will be discussed in this chapter. One of the most valuable of these rights is that these policies are guaranteed renewable. That is, once you buy a policy, that company cannot cancel your policy, for example, just because you become ill.

The downside to Medigap is that you pay the whole premium, and it is expensive. Always be aware that there is tremendous variation in the price you pay for Medigap policies even when the benefits are exactly the same. Many times the company you first think of buying from will have a premium that is 50 percent or 100 percent more than another company from which you could get identical benefits. Once you have decided what coverage you want, shop by price.

Medicare provides an up-to-date booklet entitled, *Choosing a Medigap Policy: A Guide to Health Insurance for People with Medicare.* You can get a copy by calling Medicare or going to the Medicare website.

For those of you who will be buying Medigap policies that go into effect in June of 2010 or later, a recent law has changed much of the current Medigap structure. This new structure is explained in section **11.** of this chapter.

1. Medigap SELECT Policies

The way Medigap SELECT policies work is that you must use hospitals and physicians that are affiliated with your Medigap insurance company to get its payment in full. This restricts your choice of provider from the Medigap point of view, but this means this type of policy can be significantly less expensive than other policies.

The downside to this type of policy is that it is a sort of amalgam between completely fee-for-service (Medicare part) and a restricted, managed care part (Medigap part), which can cause difficulties and misunderstandings.

If you currently have a Medicare SELECT policy, you also have the right to switch, at any time, to any regular Medigap policy being sold by the same company. The Medigap policy you switch to must have equal or less coverage than the Medicare SELECT policy you currently have.

2. Medigap Structure and Benefits

You should understand that the Medigap policies only supplement, extend, or fill in the gaps of Medicare. These policies don't pay for whole classes of care that Medicare does not cover, so none of the policies cover long-term care, routine dental or vision care, hearing aids, and prescription drugs. Note that if both you and your spouse need a policy, both of you have to get one. (In some rare cases, couples may get a small discount if you both get one from the same company.)

The best way to understand Medigap policies is to look at Table 15, which shows the standard policies and what they do and do not cover. If you live in Massachusetts, Minnesota, or Wisconsin, what follows about the structure of the policies does not apply to you. See section **3.** for more information on these states.

As you will notice from Table 15, Policy A has the least benefits, while Policy J has almost all the benefits.

Any given lettered policy is exactly the same no matter which insurance company sells it. For example, Policy E from Amalgamated Health and Accident Company has exactly the same benefits as a Policy E from Consolidated Life and Limb Limited. The policies are standard by federal law. No deviations are allowed. The only difference between policies is the cost and the service you get from the company. The best advice is to go for the lowest cost policy from a company that you think will treat you well.

The following sections discuss the benefit categories so you know exactly what they include. You should be following the chart across as you read the following sections to get a better idea of how the benefits tend to increase through the Medigap alphabet. To make this easier, you may want to print the Medigap Standard Policies Worksheet provided on the CD. The worksheet on the CD is slightly different from the standard form because it provides areas for you to write down information when looking for a policy.

2.1 Basic benefits

The basic benefit pays for your share of Part A hospital inpatient coinsurance days. These are the days beginning with your 61st day as a hospital inpatient, up to your 90th day. If you have your lifetime reserve days available and elect to use them, you have an additional 60 days. The basic benefit will also pay in full for an additional 365 days of inpatient hospital care in your lifetime. You will still be responsible for the inpatient deductible during this time, however, which was $1,100 in 2010.

The basic benefit will pay all Part B coinsurance and co-payment amounts after you pay for the yearly Part B deductible, which is $155 in 2010. It will also pay your blood deductible so you don't have to pay for, or replace, the first three pints of blood you use in any calendar year.

The basic benefit will not pay for the Part A and Part B deductibles, or Skilled Nursing Facility co-payments, or Part B excess charges; that is, the amounts you can be charged over and above the Medicare approved amount by non-participating doctors and providers. You can also get a sense of what the basic benefit doesn't

TABLE 15
MEDIGAP STANDARD POLICIES

Policies	A	B	C	D	E	F	F-Hi	G	H	I	J	J-Hi	K	L
Special notes	Basic		Very popular			Very popular	You pay first $2,000 (in 2010)				Most benefits	You pay first $2,000 (in 2010)	After you pay $4,620 (in 2010), Catastrophic begins and pays all	After you pay $2,310 (in 2010), Catastrophic begins and pays all
Basic Benefits Coinsurance for inpatient hospital days 61–90 ($275 each in 2010) Lifetime Reserve Days (up to 60) ($550 each in 2010); Payment in full for 365 additional inpatient hospital days; 20% coinsurance for Part B services after Part B deductible met; First 3 deductible pints of blood in a calendar year (Part A or B)	Yes	Yes	Yes	Yes	Yes	Yes	Yes	Yes	Yes	Yes	Yes	Yes	Yes 100% of the inpatient items, but only 50% of the Part B coinsurance * and blood deductible.	Yes 100% of the inpatient items, but only 75% of the Part B coinsurance * and blood deductible.
Part A Inpatient Deductible $1,100 in 2010 for each episode of care	No	Yes	Yes	Yes	Yes	Yes	Yes	Yes	Yes	Yes	Yes	Yes	Yes (50%)	Yes (75%)
Skilled Nursing Facility Coinsurance for days 21–100 of a covered stay – $137.50 for each day in 2010	No	No	Yes	Yes	Yes	Yes	Yes	Yes	Yes	Yes	Yes	Yes	Yes (50%)	Yes (75%)
Part B Deductible $155 in 2010	No	No	Yes	No	No	Yes	Yes	No	No	No	Yes	Yes	No	No
Part B Excess Charges Charges between 100% and 115% of Medicare's approved amount	No	No	No	No	No	Yes	Yes	Yes (80%)	No	Yes	Yes	Yes	No	No
At-Home Recovery After covered Home Health Agency visits, up to $40 a visit for 40 extra visits; max of $1,600 per calendar year; visits can't exceed number of covered visits	No	No	No	Yes	No	No	No	Yes	No	Yes	Yes	Yes	No	No
Foreign Travel Emergency 80% during the first 2 months of the trip after a $250 deductible; lifetime max of $50,000	No	No	Yes	Yes	Yes	Yes	Yes	Yes	Yes	Yes	Yes	Yes	No	No
Extra Preventive Care $120 annual maximum for extra preventative services not covered by Medicare	No	No	No	No	Yes	No	No	No	No	No	Yes	Yes	No	No
Hospice coinsurance For drugs and respite care	No	No	No	No	No	No	No	No	No	No	No	No	Yes (50%)	Yes (75%)

*Note: Policies K and L will pay 100% of the Part B coinsurance on Medicare covered preventative services.

pay for by reviewing the other policies and seeing what they do pay for. Note that all policies include the basic benefit.

2.2 Part A inpatient deductible

The Part A inpatient deductible was $1,100 in 2010. You can expect this total to rise every year. You may also pay more depending on the number of episodes of care you may need in a given year. Note that all policies except A include this category.

2.3 Skilled Nursing Facility

The Skilled Nursing Facility coinsurance is the amount you pay for each Medicare covered day of care after you have been in a Skilled Nursing Facility for 20 days. The coinsurance in 2010 was $137.50 a day for the 80 days following the end of your 20 day coverage period. All policies from C to L have this benefit. Note that in any given year only about 5 percent of beneficiaries get Skilled Nursing Facility care, and the average length of a stay is 35 days.

2.4 Part B deductible

The Part B annual deductible Is $155 in 2010 and it increases every year. You only have to pay this deductible once a calendar year. Only policies C, F, and J pay for the Part B deductible.

2.5 Part B excess charges

Part B excess charges is the amount that non-participating physicians who do not accept assignment on your claim may charge you over and above the Medicare approved amount. As was discussed in Chapter 4, this cannot be more than 15 percent above the Medicare approved amount. The limiting charge does apply to certain other Medicare covered diagnostic and radiation procedures and providers other than physicians, including ambulatory surgical centers

and physical and occupational therapists. Only Policies F, G, I, and J have excess charge coverage, while G will pay only 80 percent of the excess charge.

2.6 At-home recovery

The at-home recovery benefit is an extension of the Medicare Home Health Agency benefit. This helps to pay for additional home health agency visits after Medicare stops covering these. These visits will not be so much for therapeutic reasons, but instead for assisting you with the activities of daily living while you get better. Policies D, G, I, and J include the at-home recovery benefit.

There are many limits to this extra benefit. It will cover up to the number of visits that Medicare paid for, but will not pay for additional visits. It will cover visits only in the eight weeks after Medicare stops visiting, but no longer than eight weeks. The benefit will pay up to $40 a visit, and you will have to pay the rest. It will pay no more than $1,600 in a calendar year, which means that would be no more than 40 visits at $40 per visit. It may help to know that between 5 and 10 percent of beneficiaries get Home Health Agency visits in a given year, and that these beneficiaries get an average of 27 visits. Note that Medicare only covers those intensive levels of care, and you may want the help that this less intense level provides, especially because most people prefer to recover from an illness in their own home.

2.7 Foreign travel emergency

The foreign travel emergency benefit is included in all policies C through J and pays for 80 percent of the medical care received outside the US during the first 60 days of any trip you take, after you pay a $250 per trip deductible. It also has a $50,000 lifetime maximum. Please understand that this pays only for emergency care, and it will only pay for care that Medicare would ordinarily pay for. For example, this benefit won't cover repatriation services such as flying you back to the US in an air ambulance. You may want to consider individual trip insurance for this if you find that service desirable.

2.8 Preventive care

Preventive care pays for up to $120 per year for Medicare non-covered routine physicals or other physician-ordered health screenings Medicare does not cover. Only Policies E and J include this benefit.

2.9 High deductible policies

Both Policies F and J have the regular, normal lettered policies, but each also has a high deductible option. (Note that in Table 15 the high deductible policies are shown as F-Hi and J-Hi where Hi means High Deductible so you can tell them apart from their normal lettered counterparts of F and J.) The high deductible versions of these benefits have the exact same coverage as the regular letter counterparts, but you have to pay the first $2,000 (in 2010) before the policy pays anything. Meaning, these policies won't pay anything until you have incurred expenses that they would otherwise pay up to that $2,000. Remember that the deductible usually increases every year by the general medical inflation rate. Both the regular and high deductibles of these have the foreign travel benefit with its separate $250 deductible, which does not count toward these policies' annual deductible.

The premiums offer substantial savings. The F-Hi policy can cost less than half of what a regular F does, and the J-Hi, almost half of a regular J. Fs are very popular policies, and Js have the most coverage of all policies. Remember that the sum of $167 per month was the 2010 deductible of these policies divided by 12 months; this may

help you do some comparison shopping between the regular and high deductible options.

2.10 Catastrophic policies

Policies K and L are different because their benefits are not standard compared to the others, and, more importantly, you are required to pay on the deductibles and coinsurances on almost all Medicare covered services. (The exception being that Policies K and L will pay in full hospital inpatient coinsurances.) This is because these policies were designed to make you be more careful of medical costs so you will almost always have to pay something for a service. These policies have an annual catastrophic limit, which, once you reach it, they pay in full for all covered items, except for Part B excess charges.

Be aware that by law these amounts for the catastrophic coverage (i.e., the amount you pay out-of-pocket before the policies begin to pay in full on everything except the Part B excess charges) may change every calendar year. This is because they are indexed to Medicare inflation and they will usually increase every year. The catastrophic amounts for 2010 were $4,620 for the K policy and $2,310 for the L policy.

The major difference between these two policies is that under policy L, you pay half of what Medicare doesn't pay, and it pays the other half (i.e., 50 percent each). Under K, you pay only 25 percent and the policy pays 75 percent. The exceptions are that neither pays any of your Part B deductible or excess charges; however, both pay in full on the 365 hospital extra lifetime reserve days that all Medigap policies provide for, and they pay all your coinsurance on preventative services.

The following two sections explain how Policies K and L work. To help you a little more, see Table 16, which compares these two types

TABLE 16
HOW PLANS K AND L DIFFER FROM THE STANDARD MEDIGAP PLANS

Benefit	Plans A – J	Plan K	Plan L
Out-of-pocket maximum (in 2010)	Does not apply	$4,620	$2,310
Part A deductible	Plans B – J: 100%	50%	75%
Part A coinsurance days 61 – 90	100%	100%	100%
Part A coinsurance lifetime reserve days 91 – 150	100%	100%	100%
365 additional hospital days	100%	100%	100%
Hospice coinsurance	0%	50%	75%
Skilled Nursing Facility care coinsurance days 21 – 100	Plans C – J: 100%	50%	75%
Blood deductible	100%	50%	75%
Part B deductible	Plans C, F, J: 100%	0%	0%
Part B coinsurance	Plans C, F, J: 100%	50%*	75%*
Part B excess charges	Plans F, I, J: 100% Plan G: 80%	0%**	0%**

*K and L do pay all the Part B coinsurance on preventative services.
**Excess charges do not apply toward meeting the annual out-of-pocket maximum catastrophic limit.

of policies to the other, more standard Medigap policies.

2.10a Catastrophic policies and Part A benefits

Both Policies K and L fully cover your inpatient hospital coinsurance. These are the days beginning with your 61st day as a hospital inpatient up to your 90th day and, if you have them available, your lifetime reserve days — an additional 60 days. Once you have depleted all those days, these policies pay, in full, for an additional 365 days of inpatient hospital care in your lifetime; in other words, you will get 100 percent payment in full for an added year's worth of extra lifetime reserve days.

Both K and L will help with the inpatient deductible from the first dollar. For 2010, K pays half of the deductible (i.e., $550) and you pay the other half; L pays for 75 percent of it (i.e., $825), and you pay 25 percent (i.e., $275).

Both K and L will help pay your Skilled Nursing Facility coinsurance, which in 2010 was $137.50 a day for days 21 through 100. (Note that Medicare always pays 100 percent of the first 20 days.) Specifically, K will pay up to half of this (i.e., $68.75) a day, and you will pay the same. L will pay 75 percent (i.e., up to $103.13 a day), and you will pay the remainder (i.e., $34.37).

Both will pay, from the first dollar, their share of the first three pints of blood you use; that is, K will pay 50 percent, and you will pay 50 percent, while L will pay 75 percent, and you will pay 25 percent. This is true even if the blood expense was incurred under Part B.

Unlike any other Policy, both Policies K and L will pay on your hospice coinsurance and co-payments under Part A. Again, K will pay half and L will pay 75 percent.

2.10b Catastrophic policies and Part B benefits

After you have met the Part B deductible (i.e., $155 in 2010), both Policies K and L pay for all of the coinsurance on any Part B preventative service. These policies also pay part of the 20 percent coinsurance applicable to all other Part B services. Specifically, K pays half of your share of the coinsurance, which is 10 percent of the total allowed charge. L pays three-quarters of the coinsurance, which is 15 percent of the total allowed charge. For example, if you have a K policy, you will be responsible for 10 percent of the allowed charge, and with an L policy you will be responsible for 5 percent. For both policies, they never cover any excess charges, and the excess charges do not count towards the substantial annual deductibles.

3. Medigap Structure for Massachusetts, Minnesota, and Wisconsin

Residents in Massachusetts, Minnesota, and Wisconsin have a different structure for Medigap policies than the federal mandate. This is because these states enacted Medigap protections before the federal government, and so they were allowed to keep their laws structuring Medigap policies. One similarity to the structures in section 2. is that Wisconsin does allow companies to sell the standard catastrophic policies K and L, so for more information on these policies, read section 2.10.

Note that each of these three states has a booklet that gives more details than contained here on their Medigap plans. You may want to get the booklet for your state because it will describe mandated benefits unique to your state.

You will note that Massachusetts has only two policy types, which are basic (Core) and expanded (Supplement). Minnesota also has two, which are Basic and Extended. Wisconsin has just one, which is Basic. Table 17 is a summary of each state's structure.

In Minnesota and Wisconsin, you are allowed to pick and choose individually priced options to enhance your policy. You can add the optional riders or coverage on a one-by-one basis and tailor your Medigap policy to your specific needs and concerns. You should definitely call your state insurance commissioner's consumers' phone line or go on its website for more detailed information on these policies, or contact your State Health Insurance Assistance Program (SHIP).

Note that in Massachusetts and Minnesota, state laws require physicians to take assignment so you are generally not subject to Part B excess charges in those states. Minnesota cautions its beneficiaries not to opt for Part B excess charges unless they travel out of state.

You should be aware that both Minnesota and Wisconsin have Medigap SELECT options, while Massachusetts does not.

4. Variations in Policy Pricing

There are variations in Medigap policy pricing due to health conditions, gender, whether you are a smoker, and age. Many discussions you'll read about Medigap give you the explanation of how Medigap policies are priced according to age. The three terms used to talk about pricing by age include the following:

Community-rated: This is also known as no-age-rated, which means that every policy holder, regardless of age, pays the same premium. Therefore, your premiums will not increase because you get older, but only because of medical inflation. You will notice that some states require

TABLE 17
MEDIGAP STRUCTURE FOR MASSACHUSETTS, MINNESOTA, AND WISCONSIN

	Massachusetts		Minnesota		Wisconsin
Policy Name:	Core	Supplement 1	Basic	Extended	Basic
Hospital inpatient coinsurance (in 2010, $275 for days 61 – 90 of a stay and $550 for each of 60 lifetime reserve days)	Yes	Yes	Yes	Yes	Yes
Blood (first 3 pints per calendar year)	Yes	Yes	Yes	Yes	Yes
365 extra inpatient hospital days per lifetime	Yes	Yes	No	No	No
Part A inpatient deductible (in 2010, $1,100)	No	Yes	Opt	Yes	Opt
Skilled Nursing Facility coinsurance (in 2010, $137.50 each for days 21 – 100 of a stay)	No	Yes	Yes	Yes	Yes
Part B deductible (in 2010, $155)	No	Yes	Opt	Yes	Opt
Part B coinsurance/co-pays*	Yes	Yes	Yes	Yes	Yes
Mental health hospital extra inpatient days	60 per cal. year	120 per spell of illness	No	No	175 lifetime
Medicare non-covered Skilled Nursing Facility care (30 days)	No	No	No	No	Yes
At-home recovery (40 additional home health visits)	No	No	Opt	Yes	Yes
Extended home health care (total of 365 visits)	No	No	No	No	Opt
Part B excess charges	No	No	Opt	80%	Opt
Catastrophic coverage (pays 100% after you pay $1,000 out-of-pocket)	No	No	No	Yes	No
Preventive care	No	No	Opt	Yes	No
Foreign travel emergency	No	Yes	80%	80%	Opt
Extra foreign coverage	No	No	No	80%	No
State mandated benefits	Yes	Yes	Yes	Yes	Yes

*This also pays the Part B outpatient mental health coinsurance of 50 percent.

that premiums be set this way. In general, these policies are pricey when you first join them, but you are protected from the age-related increases.

Issue-age-rated: This means that you pay the going premium for the age you are when you first buy the policy, but from then on, the premiums increase only because of medical inflation — age is not a factor on premium increases. You lock in a price depending on how old you are when you first buy the policy. Where not mandated, few insurance companies use this approach.

Attained-age-rated: This term means that your premium is based on how old you are no matter when you originally bought the policy, with the premiums increasing as you age. For example, you will pay less for your policy at age 65 than you will when you are 70.

If you are in a state where you have the choice between an attained-age-rated policy, a community-rated, or an issue-age-rated, you have a decision to make. You may decide to buy an attained-age-rated policy, which will allow you to pay low premiums now and have the premiums escalate as you get older. Alternatively, you may choose to buy one of the other two policies (e.g., a community-rated or an issue-age-rated) and lock in a constant price for as long as you have Medigap.

In order to decide on the age-related policy, you may want to consider your life expectancy. The average life expectancy for females is 84; for males, 82. This means that you should expect to survive for another 17 to 19 years after you turn 65 at least! Community-rated and issue-age-rated policies are attractive for this reason.

The second thing to consider is the price. You can probably expect to pay from 25 to 35 percent more for an attained-age rated policy at age 75 compared to 65, and perhaps around 60 percent more at age 85. If you were to buy a community-rated policy, your initial policy at age 65 would be about 20 percent more than for an attained-age-rated policy. Premiums for each policy would be about even at age 72 or 73.

You should also be aware that in addition to variations that can occur if a state permits different types of pricing, the premiums for policies can vary for a number of reasons. Some states permit variation in price based on where you live in the state. Sometimes this is done by zip code or by county, while some states vary both by county and zip code.

Some policies vary the price depending on if you are a smoker or a nonsmoker. When buying a policy, you should be honest about this issue — remember that misrepresenting yourself is one reason an insurance company might legitimately drop you. In such an event, you would lose the right to join another Medigap policy. If you are paying a smoker's premium and you quit smoking, you should ask if you can have your premium reduced.

Many policies vary price by gender, with females paying less than males, generally by about 4 percent or less. Sometimes a particular company's policy will charge the same price regardless of gender, so a male may want to look for one of these. Sometimes these are called unisex prices.

Some Medigap policies require you to submit your claims to your Medigap insurance company. Normally, whenever Medicare processes a claim, and it knows you have a Medigap policy, it automatically crosses your claim over. In other words, Medicare makes the Medicare payment on the claim, and then electronically transmits your claim to your Medigap insurance company, which, in turn, sends its payment directly to the doctor or hospital. Basically this means you don't get involved at all in the payment process. However, be careful; not all Medigap policies work this way. Some policies require that you submit your claim to Medigap after Medicare has taken action on its part. The ones that require you to send in your own claims can sometimes be less expensive than those that do this automatically.

If you do get one of the non-crossover Medigap policies that does not automatically pay claims after Medicare does, you do have one protection. If your doctor participates in Medicare (i.e., always accepts assignment), the doctor's office is required to submit your claim to the Medicare Administrative Contractor with your Medigap policy information, and your Medigap insurance company will pay the doctor directly as soon as it knows what Medicare paid on the claim. You will be spared some paperwork if you use participating doctors.

Note that extra charges may be levied on you in some states where companies are permitted to charge you a one-time fee for applying for their policy — $25 seems to be the average rate.

5. Information gathering

Perhaps the best way for you to decide which policy to buy is for you to find out what companies offer policies in your state, and at which price for each letter policy. Most state departments of insurance (or their equivalent) have this information on their websites. You can access every state's website by going to the National Association of Insurance Commissioners website (www.naic.org), clicking on "States and Jurisdictions," and then on your state. Once on your state's website, you need to find the section on Medicare, Medicare Supplement Insurance, or Medigap.

Some sites give you detailed information on why the prices for a particular policy vary; some don't. Many break down the cost of the policy by age ranges (e.g., 65, 75, 85). Some mix individual policies and group policies together; and, sometimes, they mix in the SELECT policies with the regular ones. Some sites may mix the high and low options together under the F and J policies, rather than showing these in completely separate categories. You also need to pay attention to the name of the insurance companies carefully, because many of them look alike (e.g., Continental General Insurance Company is not Continental Life Insurance Company).

If you don't find the information you are looking for on the website, call your state insurance office and ask that the information be sent to you. The contact information for the state departments of insurance is included in the Resources section on the CD.

Use the Medigap Standard Policies Worksheet (included on the CD) to record the information you find about different policies. This will help you keep organized while you are sorting through the various policies and their cost variations. On the worksheet there is a place for you to write down the number of companies offering a policy. If only a few companies offer a particular letter policy, it may be a signal to you that there is not a lot of competition, and you need to look closely at the prices to see if you are getting a good or bad deal for that particular letter policy.

Note that some companies require you to pay quarterly instead of monthly, and they show their premiums in quarterly amounts. If needed, be sure you convert that quarterly premium into a monthly figure if the other companies' quotes are in months. If you are interested in a SELECT policy, use a separate sheet to write this information down, so you can compare the regular policies and the SELECT policies separately.

Once you have written the prices down, you will see that there is a lot of variability in the price, which is extremely important to know. Recall that you get the same thing in each lettered policy, no matter who sells it.

Don't hesitate to seek advice from others. It may help you to talk to someone such as a State Health Insurance Assistance Program (SHIP) counselor who has experience with the policies available in your area. Contact information for SHIP is included in the Resources on the CD.

5.1 Finding the policy that works for you

You'll notice in your research that there are more A policies offered than any other. This is because if a company wants to sell any policy, it's got to offer an A policy. You should note that recently the most popular policies have been C and the regular F. These policies, both of which roughly cost about 60 percent more than the basic A, have a good number of benefits — you may want to consider them for a good balance of premium cost and benefits.

Policy A has the fewest benefits and is the least comprehensive. However, it is the least expensive of the standard policies. You might want to consider an A policy only if you can afford to pay out-of-pocket for many medical expenses.

Policy B adds the Part A hospital inpatient deductible to the Policy A benefits, which was $1,100 in 2010. These policies cost about $40 a month (or about $500 per year) more than an A policy. Considering you may have to pay the $1,100 deductible more than once in a year, and even if it happens only once, that's still a lot of money to pay at one time, so the additional money you pay for this letter seems pretty reasonable.

Policy C will cost you about $20 to $30 per month more than policy B. This is because C pays your B deductible, but the deductible is only $155. Even though these are popular policies, unless you can get a really good price for one (and you might as there is so much variability), you should consider another policy.

The C and H policies cover the exact same thing except H does not pay the Part B deductible. You should never pay more than $13 extra a month for a C over an H (i.e., 2010 deductible of $155 divided by 12 months).

You may want to look at policies D, E, or H, which don't pay the deductible but have the benefits shown in Table 15 and both of which seem to be priced only $10 or $15 a month more than policy B. You might want to consider D if you have no other source for at-home recovery, but if you do, you might want to go for E. If neither of these feels right for you, join H. Note that policies D, E, and H do not pay for excess charges, so you may want to get one of these policies only if you have a doctor that takes assignment or if you live in a state where assignment is mandatory.

Note that some H policies, which have fewer benefits than D or E, sell for more. This reiterates that the prices of these policies are not always rational and indeed vary tremendously. Remember that just because a policy has a higher letter doesn't mean it's always better. If you are talking to an agent who is trying to sell you an H, which costs more than a D or E, try a different company.

If you are worried about excess charges, you should consider F, G, I, or J, which pay the excess charges; G pays only 80 percent of the excess charge. Policies I and G are identical except that policy I pays 100 percent of the excess charges, so G should cost less than I in premiums. F is the same but it also pays your Part B deductible and, as with policy C, this makes it pricey for what you get.

J is the deluxe policy with everything and it's also the most expensive; keep that in mind when trying to get a feel for prices.

Now that we've covered the basic letter policies A through J, we need to talk about the two policies that have the high deductible option. The high deductible means a deductible where you have to pay the first $2,000 (in 2010) in expenses before your Medigap pays anything. This amount is indexed to the US urban consumer price index, and so it goes up almost every calendar year by the general rate of inflation. You will pay a lot of money before your policy pays anything, but your premiums will be a lot less. If you can come up with the cash for the deductible, you might want to look for one of these high deductible policies with a low premium.

The high deductible option costs about a third of the regular F option, so you can save a lot on premiums. The spread between a regular J and a high deductible J does not seem to be as good, but again, you need to look at the specific prices available to you. One way to consider it is that you will have to pay $167 a month in medical costs before a high deductible policy pays anything (i.e., the $167 is the 2010 annual deductible of $2,000 divided by 12).

6. Discounts

You should inquire about discounts or reductions on the premiums you have to pay for your policy. While only a few companies offer discounts, some will give you a discount if both you and your spouse buy a Medigap policy from them. Some companies will do so if you agree to pay by electronic funds transfer, meaning they withdraw your premium payments monthly from your bank account. Some will give you a discount if you pay your annual premium all at once. First, choose which policy is the best for you and then ask about discounts as you want to get the policy that fits you best with the lowest premium.

7. Underwriting

You should also be aware that insurance companies can require underwriting when they sell you a Medigap policy if your state permits this. Underwriting occurs when the insurer has you answer questions about your health, requires you to take a physical exam, and/or looks at your medical records. Sometimes a company will use this method to price your premium. You may be able to get a better deal with a company that does this if you are quite healthy. However, a company may decide not to sell you a policy if it's not sure you're healthy, but it can't do this if you have a right to a policy, as explained in section 8.

7.1 Preexisting conditions

Even though a company must sell you a Medigap policy when you are in the open enrollment period, it may require that you serve a preexisting condition period, if your state allows this. For example, if you have diabetes, the policy would not pay for any diabetes-related treatments or supplies during a certain period. The maximum time that it can impose this condition on you is six months. It cannot impose this on you if you had creditable insurance for the six months before you had your policy. If you had creditable insurance for some but not all of those six months, it must subtract the length of its waiting period by the number of months you had that insurance.

Creditable coverage for Medigap purposes means just about any health insurance you had, such as an Employer (or Union) Group Health Plan or a health insurance policy you had yourself. Insurance that doesn't count are limited policies such as those for dental or vision care, hospital indemnity insurance (you typically get so many dollars per hospital stay or per day in the hospital), disease insurance (e.g., cancer insurance), and long-term care policies.

Note that genetic testing or information cannot be gathered or used to deny or impose a condition of issuing or pricing a Medigap policy.

8. Medigap Rights and Protections

You have a number of rights under federal law when it comes to Medigap and this section will help explain those rights.

8.1 Your Medigap open enrollment period

You have the right to buy a Medigap policy in your Medigap open enrollment period. This is the six months after you turn age 65 and are enrolled in Medicare Part B; that is, your enrollment period begins the first day of the month in the month during which you turn 65. This is also the beginning of your Part B entitlement. However, if you worked past age 65 and had a good Employer Group Health Plan and took Part A but did not want Part B, you may not have signed up for Medigap or Part B at 65. If you now retire at 68, for example, and lose your employer plan, you may sign up for Part B, and your Medigap open enrollment period will begin the first day of the month that you have Part B.

It could be that you are a disabled or an end-stage renal disease beneficiary and have had Part B for many years, and now you turn 65. Your Medigap open enrollment period will begin on the first day of the month you turn 65.

Once you go into your Medigap open enrollment period, it cannot be changed. It's very important for you to buy a policy in these six months. This is because every Medigap insurance company offering policies where you live —

- must sell you any Medigap insurance policy it offers;

- cannot charge you more for your policy if you have health problems; and

- cannot make you wait for your coverage to start, except it may make you wait for up to six months for a preexisting condition you have before you are covered for it.

8.2 Your special guaranteed issue rights

In addition to your Medigap open enrollment period right, you also have an array of nine special guaranteed issue rights that make sure you can get a Medigap policy when certain events happen. These are a varied set of rights to protect you if you have a Medigap policy and lose it.

Before discussing your rights you need to understand the following important points:

- You need to carefully observe the time frames for these rights, which are mostly shorter than the six months you get for your Medigap open enrollment period. Basically, you'll have only 63 calendar days to apply for your Medigap after your other coverage ends.

- Note that in many situations you may not have access to every policy in your state; the most common policies are A, B, C, F, F-High, K, or L.

- You should exercise your rights quickly, meaning you should apply for a Medigap policy as soon as you can so that you won't have a break in coverage.

- The events that cause you to lose your coverage tend to involve significant changes and even disconnects in your health-care delivery system (e.g., you might be moving to another state, leaving managed care to go to Original Medicare, or retiring from your job) so you need to keep a paper trail of what goes on in order to protect your rights. Save all paperwork you receive and the postmarked envelopes the paperwork comes in. Also copy any letter or application you send, and mail "return receipt requested" so that you can demonstrate what happened and protect your rights.

- Your state may have wider rights than these federal ones, so it's always worth checking out your state's rights.

The following paragraphs discuss your nine special guaranteed rights in detail:

1. **Your Medigap policy terminates because of no fault of yours.** This may because the insurance company went bankrupt or it stopped doing business in your state. If so, you have a right to buy Medigap policies A, B, C, F, F-High, K, or L from any company that sells these in your area. You must apply for your new policy within 63 calendar days from the date your old Medigap policy ends. The best time to apply is as soon as you get notice of the termination, to keep your coverage seamless.

2. **You terminate your Medigap policy because your insurance company hasn't followed its rules or because it misled you.** If your insurance company is not paying your claims as it should, or it told you it would cover things it won't, or there was deception on the company's part, you can file a written grievance or protest with your state insurance commissioner and try to get a ruling that your insurance company is at fault and that you have a right to leave it. (You should specifically ask for this right in your grievance or protest letter.) If you win the ruling, you will have a right to buy Medigap policies A, B, C, F, F-High, K, or L from any company that sells these in your area. You have to apply for your new Medigap policy within 63 calendar days of the day your coverage ends on your old policy. You shouldn't drop your policy until you get a favorable ruling from your insurance commissioner.

3. **You have an Employer (or Union) Group Health Plan or a Consolidated Omnibus Budget Reconciliation Act (COBRA) plan, and it is ending.** Your plan must be paying as a secondary payer, meaning your medical bills are paid first by Medicare and then by your plan. In order to get this right, your participation in the plan must be ending through no fault of your own; for example, your employer goes out of business or stops offering the plan. (Note that if you fail to pay your premiums or voluntarily drop your coverage, this right does not apply.) If this is your situation, you have the guaranteed issue right to buy Medigap policies A, B, C, F, F-High, K, or L from any company that sells these in your area. You must apply for a Medigap policy within 63 calendar days of the latest of the date —

- your coverage actually ends,

- on your notice that your coverage is ending, or

- on a claim denial notice if this is how you first discover that your coverage has ended.

You can get COBRA because your Employer (or Union) Group Health Plan ends and you need a new health plan. If you are a Medicare beneficiary when your Employer Group Health Plan ends, you can, at this point get either COBRA or a Medigap policy. However, your COBRA will usually end, so it is better to sign up for Medigap in the first place.

4. **You join a Medicare Advantage Plan when you are first eligible for Medicare at age 65.** If you decide, within a year of joining your Medicare Advantage Plan, that you don't like it and want to go into Original Medicare, you have the right to buy any Medigap policy in your area. Note that you have to give your managed care plan notice that you want to disenroll, and your disenrollment date must be before you have been in the plan for a full 12 months. Once you give notice to your plan, you have 60 calendar days before your disenrollment date to 63 calendar days after you disenroll to buy a Medigap policy.

5. **You are in Original Medicare and you have a Medigap policy.** Suppose you decide to try a Medicare Advantage or managed care plan for the very first time, so you join a plan and leave your Medigap policy. Within a year, you decide you don't like your new arrangement and want to return to Original Medicare. You have the right to buy the exact same Medigap policy you dropped when you went into the Medicare Advantage Plan. As in number 4, you have to give notice to your plan and the date to disenroll must be before you have been in the plan for a full 12 months. Once you have given notice, you have 60 calendar days before your disenrollment date to 63 calendar days after you disenroll to repurchase the same policy you had before from the same company. If this company does not offer the same policy, you have the guaranteed right to Medigap policy A, B, C, F, F-High, K, or L but from any insurance company that offers it in your area.

6. **Your Medicare Advantage Plan terminates you because it stops operating in your area.** If your Medicare Advantage Plan goes bankrupt or it stops doing business where you live, you will get a letter from your plan discussing its termination, and telling you that you have the right to switch to another Medicare Advantage Plan in your area. You also have a right to buy Medigap policy A, B, C, F, F-High, K, or L from any company that sells these in your area if you decide Medicare managed care is not for you. In this situation, you have two different opportunities to leave your plan and get a Medigap policy:

   - When you receive the letter advising you that your plan is terminating, you can disenroll from it right away. You have 63 calendar days from the day you actually are disenrolled from it to get a Medigap policy.

   - You can wait until the actual date your plan stops. You will automatically be put into Original Medicare on that date, and from that point you have 63 calendar days to purchase your Medigap policy.

7. **Your move from your service area of your Medicare Advantage Plan.** You must legally reside in the service area in which the Medicare program contracts with a Medicare Advantage Plan to operate. If you move away, the place you move to may not be covered by your current plan. In this case, you must disenroll from your plan. If you don't join another plan, you have a right to buy a Medigap policy A, B, C, F, F-High, K, or L from any company that sells these in your new

area. You may apply for your new policy as early as 60 days before your actual disenrollment date from your plan, and you have only 63 calendar days from that date to apply for your Medigap policy.

8. **You leave your Medicare Advantage Plan because your plan hasn't followed its rules or because it misled you.** If you can show that the Medicare Advantage Plan is not giving you the care it should, not paying your claims as it should, not covering services it said it would, or there was deception on the plan's part, you can file a written grievance or protest with your state insurance commissioner and/or with the Centers for Medicare & Medicaid Services and try to get a ruling that your plan is at fault and that you have a right to leave it. (You should specifically ask for this right in your grievance or protest letter.) If you get a determination in your favor, you have the right to join any Medigap insurer in your area and buy an A, B, C, F, F-High, K, or L Medigap policy. You have to give a disenrollment notice to your plan and, once you do so, you have 60 calendar days before your disenrollment date to 63 calendar days after your disenrollment to buy a Medigap policy.

9. **You are in Original Medicare and you have a Medigap policy.** You decide to try a Medigap SELECT policy for the very first time so you switch from your regular Medigap to a Medigap SELECT policy. Within a year, you decide you don't like your Medigap SELECT arrangement and want to go back to a regular Medigap policy. You have the right to buy the exact same Medigap policy you disenrolled from when you went to your Medigap SELECT.

You have to give your Medigap SELECT company notice that you want to disenroll, and your disenrollment date must be before you have had the Medigap SELECT policy a full 12 months. Once you give notice to your company, you have the period of 60 calendar days before your disenrollment date to 63 calendar days after this date to repurchase the same policy you had before from the same company with which you previously had your policy. If this company does not offer the same policy, you have the guaranteed right to a Medigap policy A, B, C, F, F-High, K, or L from any insurance company that offers it in your area.

8.3 Disabled beneficiary's special suspension right

There is also a special right for a beneficiary younger than 65 who has Medicare because of a disability, but not because of end-stage renal disease. Specifically, if you are a disabled beneficiary and have a Medigap policy, and you become enrolled in an Employer (or Union) Group Health Plan, you have the right to suspend your Medigap policy. What this means is that your Medigap will no longer pay for anything effective on or after the date of suspension, but if you need to get it back, which you would probably want to do if you lost your Employer Group Health Plan, you can reactivate your account. You will pay only the premium you otherwise would have to pay when you reactivate it. You can activate it without regard to any preexisting condition.

Note that you have to specifically tell your Medigap insurer that you want to suspend the policy. You should notify the insurer in writing that you are suspending the policy. When you learn that you will no longer be covered under the Employer Group Health Plan, you should notify your insurer right away and arrange for you policy to be reactivated so that you are continuously covered. Note that you must notify your insurer within 90 calendar days of losing your group health plan.

8.4 Medicaid beneficiary's special suspension right

If you have a Medigap policy and you then become entitled to Medicaid, you probably will not need your Medigap policy since a Medicaid program will typically pay for the things covered by your Medigap policy. Therefore, you have the right to suspend your Medigap policy. When suspended, you will not have to pay the premiums for the policy and it will not pay any benefits.

You must suspend your Medigap policy within 90 days of your entitlement to Medicaid, and you can keep your policy suspended for up to 24 months. If, within this time frame, you need to restart your policy, usually because you lose your Medicaid eligibility, you can notify the insurance company, begin paying your premiums, it will immediately cover you without regard to any illness or condition you have.

8.5 Special Medigap consumer rights and protections

In addition to your open enrollment period, guaranteed issue, and suspension rights, federal law mandates a number of other protections surrounding Medigap policies. These have been classified as consumer protections and will help ensure that you are dealt with fairly and not unduly taken advantage of when buying a Medigap policy. Again, your state may have additional protections that apply specifically to Medigap policies, or more broadly to insurance

products, or to general consumer rights. If you feel you have been taken advantage of in any way, contact your state insurance commissioner.

8.5a Return of a policy

Every applicant for Medigap insurance has the right to return any policy or certificate for any reason within 30 calendar days of receiving the policy. The insurance company is required to refund all premiums and any other fees that have been paid. Your 30 days begins when you receive the policy or certificate. If you buy a policy that the agent delivers to you on the same day you complete the application (sometimes called a field-issued policy), your 30 days begins when you receive a notice in the mail from the insurer. Always document the date you received the policy and the date you return the policy to the insurance company or the agent, which you should do using "return receipt requested" mail.

8.5b Waiting periods for preexisting medical conditions

No Medigap insurance policy may ever require a waiting period longer than six months for coverage of a preexisting condition. If you replace one policy or certificate with another, and have satisfied the waiting period under the first one, the replacing insurance company may not impose a new waiting period for the same preexisting condition. You must be given credit for your prior coverage.

However, if you go from one Medigap policy to another one with more benefits than the first, the company can impose a waiting period, but only on the new benefits. For example, if you go from policy A to B (the only difference is that B will pay your inpatient hospital deductible) and if you were to be hospitalized for a preexisting condition, the policy would not pay that deductible. It would have to pay if you owned the policy at least six months prior to switching as it would be creditable coverage. Another example would be that if you owned the A policy for four months, and you were hospitalized after you had the new policy for only three months, it would pay, as your preexisting condition period would only be for two more months, and you had the policy for three months.

8.5c Right to renew for life

Your Medigap policy is guaranteed renewable, which means that you have the right to renew your Medigap policy for life. Your insurance company cannot cancel your policy because you get older or become unhealthy.

8.5d Restrictions on selling Medigap policies

If you have Medicaid, it is illegal for an insurance company to sell you a Medigap policy unless Medicaid pays your Medigap premium. If Medicaid pays your Medicare premium, deductibles, and coinsurance, you can buy Medigap policies H, I, or J. If Medicaid pays all or part of your Medicare Part B premium, you can buy any Medigap policy.

It is illegal for an insurance company to sell you a Medigap policy if you already have one. The only exception is that the company may do so if you tell it in writing that you will cancel the policy you already have.

If you are enrolled in a Medicare Advantage or managed care plan, an insurance company cannot sell you a Medigap policy because it cannot pay for your cost sharing deductibles, co-payments, or coinsurance under such a plan.

No company can tell you that its Medigap is approved by the Medicare program or by the federal government or that it is federal insurance. Medigap is private insurance you buy from an insurance company, although the company may be associated with a particular organization. No agent can say it is a Medicare representative or use the seals or logos of the Centers for Medicare & Medicaid Services or the Social Security Administration.

9. If You Kept a Medigap Policy with Drug Coverage

Certain Medigap policies (i.e., H, I, and J), purchased before 2006 included prescription drug coverage. Most beneficiaries who had these policies converted them to policies without this drug coverage and then joined Medicare Part D. Note that Part D plans usually have better coverage and lower premiums than Medigap policies with drug coverage. Part D plans are heavily subsidized by the federal government while Medigap policies with drug coverage are not.

If you decided to keep your Medigap prescription drug coverage, you should consider if you would have better coverage joining Part D. Unfortunately, your right to drop your Medigap prescription drug coverage while maintaining all the rest of the policy has expired. However, you may be able convince a Medigap insurer to sell you a policy without that coverage. You can join a Part D plan on the first of any year.

There are two different scenarios. The first is that you may have gotten a letter from your Medigap insurer telling you that your prescription drug coverage with them was credible, that is, that it was at least as good as Medicare Part D. If so, you won't have to pay a premium penalty to join a Part D plan. You may be able to find a better deal than what your Medigap policy offers. If so, you should try to convince your Medigap insurer to remove your drug coverage from your Medigap policy. Note that your insurance provider doesn't have to do this, so proceed cautiously.

If your coverage has not been creditable and you can remove your Medigap prescription drug coverage, but keep your Medigap policy, you will have to find a Part D plan that will give you a good deal. You also need to take your penalty into account. For example, if you sign up as of January 1, 2010, it would be $15.30 per month (i.e., 1 percent for each of the 48 months you were not signed up in 2006, 2007, 2008, and 2009 times the 2010 national average monthly premium of $31.94, rounded to the nearest ten cents).

10. Contacting Companies

By now you may have settled on one or two lettered policies and maybe half a dozen or fewer companies, and you'll have a general idea of what a policy will cost. When you begin contacting companies to inquire further into their policies, you will find that they want to send an agent to you. If you are not interested in going through the sales pitch, but just want information, tell them you are not ready to buy and ask them to send you information about the policies you are considering.

The "Questions to Ask When Researching Medigap Policies Worksheet""included on the CD gives you questions to ask companies when you are searching for a policy. Your general strategy should be to get the policy you can afford with the benefits you want.

11. Major Medigap Changes in June, 2010

Effective on June 1, 2010, substantial changes will be made to Medigap insurance. Plans E, H, I, J, and J-Hi will no longer be available. Not to worry for those who have one of these plans: If you enroll in one of these policies before that date, you can keep it. The new rules apply only to policies sold in June of 2010 and onward.

While A, B, C, D, F, F-Hi, K, and L will continue to be available, their benefits will be changed somewhat. Specifically, no policy will have the "at-home recovery" or the "extra preventative care" benefit. However, "hospice coinsurance" will become part of the basic benefit all policies must have.

Two new policies will be sold, which are M and N. The new policy M will be the same as the changed policy D, except that it will pay only half of your inpatient deductible, not the full amount. Policy N will be the same as the changed policy D, except that you will have to pay the first $20 of coinsurance for any physician visit, and the first $50 of any co-payment for a hospital emergency room visit (but not if you are admitted as an inpatient). All of this information is laid out in the Medigap Standard Policies Worksheet June 2010, which is included on the CD.

One other change will take place: If a company sells any Medigap policies, it will have to sell A policies (as plans must do so now), plus it will have to offer either a C or an F policy. Unfortunately, it will take some time for the new policies to be analyzed in the same way we have done in this chapter for the policies now in effect. This is just a guess, but it is likely that the C and F policies will continue to be very popular and, for that reason, somewhat competitive, so you should at least price these out when you go to shop for a Medigap policy in June of 2010 or beyond.

12. Medical Bill Tracking

As this is the first of several chapters on insurance in addition to Medicare, it seems like a good place to discuss how to keep track of your Medicare and other insurance. One of the things you need to keep track of is your medical bills.

If you get really sick, you are going to be treated by a wide variety of providers and the bills will start to compile. To help you stay organized, the CD includes the following worksheets for you to keep track of your bills:

- One Payer Bill Tracking Worksheet: Use this worksheet if you have only Medicare or you are in Medicare Advantage care.

- Two Payer Bill Tracking Worksheet: Use this worksheet if Medicare is your primary payer and you have other insurance (e.g., Medigap or retirement group health).

- Two Payer (Medicare secondary payer) Bill Tracking Worksheet: Use this worksheet if Medicare is your secondary payer and you have other insurance that is the primary payer (e.g., employee group health).

You will see item numbers in the first column of these worksheets. When you get a Medicare Summary Notice it will often have several completely unrelated services listed. I have found that if you write an item number on your doctor's bill and the same item number next to the same service on the Medicare Summary Notice

or other claims documents, that it is much easier to keep things in order. For example, your doctor's bill may only include the name of the doctor, while the Medicare Summary Notice may label the service under the clinic's name instead of the doctor's name. Another example may be that the doctor's bill you got called the service you received an "office visit," while the Medicare Summary Notice termed it as "90015 — intermediate." Using item numbers to keep services identified can be very helpful. Other than that, the forms are self-explanatory.

Even though almost all Medicare claims are assigned, there is an assignment column in which you can indicate that something was not assigned, and so you can expect to pay more for that service. Also, for simplicity, note there are no separate columns for you to keep track of deductibles as your Medicare Summary Notice will tell you how much to pay. However, if you are detail-oriented, you can use the remarks column to keep track of this.

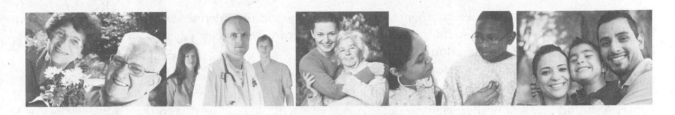

11
Medicare and Private Health Insurance: Coordinating Your Benefits

The vast majority of Medicare beneficiaries have other health insurance. This is because Medicare only pays part of their health costs.

You need to protect yourself by getting other health insurance to work with your Medicare. Besides giving you specific information on how Medicare coordinates with other health insurance programs, the basic theme of this chapter and the next chapter is to offer information on the various options, so you can develop the best strategy as you go into retirement.

On the CD you will find the Medicare Coordination of Benefits Table. You can print and keep the table with your Medicare records for quick answers to questions about primary and secondary payers when dealing with Medicare and private health insurance.

1. Coordination of Benefits

Before getting into the specifics of Medicare and the different insurance programs, you need to know how Medicare actually administers its Coordination of Benefits activities. Coordination of Benefits means the Medicare program, as well as all other insurance carriers, will

endeavor to pay only what their share of the medical bill is and never together pay more than the bill's total. As you would expect with a federal program, there are many rules and regulations to dictate how this is done.

You'll see the terms *primary* and *secondary*, which simply means who pays first and who pays second. Sometimes you'll see the term Medicare Secondary Payer, which is a somewhat misleading term Medicare often uses in talking about its Coordination of Benefits efforts. It's misleading because it sometimes describes situations in which Medicare will never pay on a claim.

Medicare employs several different contractors to help coordinate benefits; the key one is the Coordination of Benefits Contractor. It gathers information on who should be paying claims and makes sure that the Medicare Administrative Contractors know how to process claims involving more than just Medicare. If you need some information about your Coordination of Benefits or to report changes in your insurance situation, contact the Coordination of Benefits Contractor (the contact information is included in the Resources on the CD). If you need information about a specific claim or overpayment notice involving Coordination of Benefits, call Medicare. Note that the Coordination of Benefits Contractor doesn't actually process any claims or overpayment collections.

You should also know that Medicare carries out what it calls *data matching* in which it runs its databases against many others to find out if unreported third-party insurance should be paying for its claims. These databases include ones you might expect (e.g., Social Security) as well as ones you wouldn't expect (e.g., Internal Revenue Service). Its claims processing systems can figure out that some other party should be paying on a claim where it looks like an industrial illness is involved or that an accident occurred. It's important that the Coordination of Benefits Contractor has this information up front. If something happens to change your insurance situation, for example, if your spouse retires and your Employer Group Health Insurance is now on a retirement basis, report this to the Coordination of Benefits Contractor. These factors make a difference in who pays your claims first.

Note that there is a separate contractor who is in charge of dealing with claims that Medicare paid but should not have because another party is liable for the service or supply. This contractor is called the Medicare Secondary Payer Recovery Contractor. You may be contacted by this type of contractor in situations such as where your employer's insurance company should have paid, or Workers' Compensation should have paid due to an accident.

You should know that if a Medicare Secondary Payer Recovery Contractor is working on a case that involves you, and you have set up a MyMedicare account, information on the case the contractor is working on will appear under the "My MSP" tab that will appear in your MyMedicare account. As the contractor updates this information weekly, this can be helpful to you or the representative working on your Medicare Secondary Payer case.

As part of your enrollment process, Medicare will mail you an Initial Enrollment Questionnaire. When you have completed the questionnaire, you will have to send it to the Coordination of Benefits Contractor. Typically, you will get this questionnaire three months before your entitlement begins. The form has five slightly different versions; the one you get depends on how you get entitled to Medicare (e.g., turn age 65, have end-stage renal disease, etc.).

The questionnaire will ask if you are working and if your employer has employer group health coverage, whether you have coverage through your spouse's employment, and if you have any prescription drug coverage through such insurance. It also asks if any liability situation such as Workers' Compensation exists for you, and the details about this. The Coordination of Benefits Contactor's number is on the form if you need help or have any questions.

You can also complete the questionnaire by going online to your MyMedicare account. This is actually much easier because the online questionnaire skips over the questions you do not need to respond to and takes no more than two minutes to complete. Instructions on how to access this will come with your questionaire.

Another good source of information is the booklet, *Medicare and Other Health Benefits: Your Guide to Who Pays First* (publication CMS-02179), which you can get by calling Medicare.

2. Employer and Union Group Health Insurance

You need to understand that from the Medicare perspective there are two very different types of health insurance that you can get from your employer or union: insurance that you have while you or a spouse are still working, and insurance that you have after you or your spouse retire or are separated from your employer. These are both known as Employer Group Health Plans (EGHP) even though you may no longer be an employee, or you get them through a union.

2.1 Retirement employer and union group health insurance

As a Medicare beneficiary, you may have your coverage because you or you spouse retired and your former employer or union provides for coverage for its retirees. (Note that if you have your insurance through your retired spouse while you continue to work, it's still called retiree coverage.)

As you approach your retirement, you need to start investigating just what your health plan will look like when you get Medicare. If you are retired, you should know that the basic rule is that Medicare will be the primary payer of your health care, and your retirement plan will be the secondary payer. Because of this, many retirement plans are more or less tailored to fill in what Medicare does not pay for, so they may well pay for Medicare deductibles, coinsurance, and possibly excess charges. You need to find out which family members will be covered and whether or not they have Medicare. Obviously, if they have no other insurance, you will want to keep your plan.

The first thing you need to understand is what your plan will pay after Medicare has made its claims decision. You will need to consider the answers to the following questions:

- Will your plan pay your deductibles, co-insurance, and/or co-payments? If so, will it pay them all or in part? If in part, how much will be covered?

- Does your plan have prescription drug coverage? If so, is this coverage creditable or not?

- Will your plan pay for things Medicare won't, such as annual physicals, eyeglasses, dental care, and foreign travel care?

- Does your plan have catastrophic protection? If so, when does this start and what are the limits?

The next thing you have to figure out is how much you will pay for your insurance in retirement. For some of you, it will be free. In other cases, you may have to pay a premium and the premium may escalate as time goes on. You may be required to have Part B and pay those premiums yourself or your employer or union may pay all or part of them.

Finally, you have to figure out if your plan will be around for the long term. Nowadays, companies are ending their retirees' health plans because of cost, bankruptcies, corporate mergers, and buyouts. Even when this doesn't happen, you can possibly expect cost controls to reduce your benefits rather than to enhance them as time goes on.

The only way you can tell if your plan is a good deal is to talk to your human resources department or benefits administration people. Ask for your plan's benefits booklet and carefully read through it. Talk with fellow employees or union members who have retired and ask about their experiences with the plan. The best general advice is that you should always keep your retirement plan.

One reason to keep your retirement plan is that under Medicare law, a retiree's group health insurance automatically becomes the secondary payer and Medicare becomes the primary payer. All this means is that when you have a health service, the bill first gets sent to Medicare and it decides how much can be charged and how much it will pay. The remaining charge goes to your retirement plan. Many retirement plans will usually go along with Medicare's decision on how much can be charged and the retirement plan will pay the difference between what Medicare paid and what you paid. (Recall that when Medicare decides what a provider can charge you, that decision holds whether or not you have any other insurance.)

You can often get a Medicare-covered service completely paid for by Medicare and your retirement Employer Group Health Plan (EGHP). While this is not true for every retirement group plan, this is how many employer group plans work, so it's a good deal. Your plan may pay for things Medicare does not cover, which will make any particular plan an even better deal.

Remember that if your retiree EGHP has prescription coverage that is creditable under Part D, it's as good as Part D. If, later on, you must or want to get Part D, you won't have to pay any penalties on your Part D premium if you sign up if you have a retiree EGHP.

You should always be aware that if you drop your retirement plan, you may never be able to get it back. At the very least, carry it into retirement and see how it works out. If you become convinced that it's not a good option, you may want to consider something else.

2.2 Working employer and union group health insurance

You need to find out, if you decide to continue working after age 65, whether or not your employer continues to provide health insurance for its employees who get or have Medicare. If your employer has an Employer Group Health Plan (EGHP), it is required to continue to provide the insurance under federal law if it has 20 or more employees.

Note that you have some powerful protections under federal law in connection with your EGHP. If you are age 65 or older, and your plan has 20 or more employees, the benefits it offers to you can't be different than those it offers to employees younger than 65. If it offers benefits to spouses, these benefits can't be different if the spouse is older than 65. The same protection is also available to the employee of any size plan that has end-stage renal disease. The same situation applies for spouse's benefits if your spouse gets end-stage renal disease.

You need to understand that the rules on who pays first for working employee benefits are different than the rules for who pays when the insured gets retiree EGHP insurance. You don't need to know all rules, just the one that applies to you. In situations in which you, the Medicare beneficiary, are age 65 or older and you —

- have Medicare and an EGHP, are still working, and your company has 20 or more employees, your plan will be the primary payer with Medicare as the secondary payer.

- have Medicare and an EGHP, you are still working, and your company has fewer than 20 employees, Medicare will be the primary payer with your plan as the secondary payer.

- are the spouse of a person of any age who is working, you are covered under his or her EGHP, and his or her company has 20 or more employees, your spouse's plan will be the primary payer for you with Medicare as the secondary payer.

- are the spouse of a person of any age who is working, and you are covered under his or her EGHP, and his or her company has fewer than 20 employees, Medicare will be the primary payer for you with your spouse's plan as the secondary payer.

In situations in which you, the Medicare beneficiary, have Medicare because you are disabled (and younger than 65) and you are —

- covered by an EGHP from your former employer and the employer has 100 or more employees, your plan is the primary payer with Medicare as the secondary payer. The 100-or-more employee plans are sometimes referred to as Large Employer Group Health Plans. (Note: it is unusual but possible that even though you are on disability, you can get your coverage from your current employer; perhaps you are doing a trial work period to see if you have recovered enough to be able to go back to work.)

- covered by an EGHP from your former employer and the employer has less than 100 employees, Medicare will be the primary payer with your plan being the secondary payer. (As above, it is possible to get coverage from your employer.)

- the spouse of a person of any age who is working, you are covered under his or her EGHP, and his or her company has 100 or more employees, your spouse's plan will be the primary payer with Medicare being the secondary payer.

- the spouse of a person of any age who is working, you are covered under his or her EGHP, and his or her company has less than 100 employees, Medicare is the primary payer with your spouse's plan as secondary payer.

In situations in which you, the Medicare beneficiary, have or could have Medicare because you are under 65 and have end-stage renal disease, and you have an EGHP on your own or from your working spouse or parent, the plan will be the primary payer with Medicare as the secondary payer for the first 30 months of your entitlement to Medicare. This presumes you applied for and got Medicare as soon as you could.

If you could get Medicare Part A because you have end-stage renal disease, and you have an EGHP on your own or because of your working spouse or parent, the plan will be the primary payer with Medicare as the secondary payer, for the first 30 months of your potential entitlement to Medicare. Beginning with the 31st month after you could have been entitled to Medicare, your EGHP will pay only what Medicare would not pay, whether or not you have Medicare at this point.

What's going on here is that the Medicare program is limiting the liability of EGHP to paying primarily only for 30 months, whether or not you apply for Medicare. You would always want to file to get it at the 31st month. You should know that whenever you start dialysis or are on the list for a kidney transplant, that information is passed to Medicare, even though you did not apply for it. Medicare will know when your potential entitlement begins.

You should not automatically assume that the outfit that you or your spouse works for has less than 20 employees. This is because some companies, usually smaller ones, will band together with other companies to get an EGHP policy. If this happens, and any one of the companies has more than 20 people, that qualifies all the companies as having more than 20 employees. In this case, for those Medicare beneficiaries older than 65, their EGHP will be their primary payer. If any company has more than 100 employees, the plan will be considered a Large Employer Group Health Plan, and it will be the primary payer for disabled Medicare beneficiaries. It may also be that a company allows individuals to sign up with its plan, maybe a self-employed person, a board director, or a business associate. If you are or your spouse is an individual insured through an EGHP, the size of the largest company will govern.

It's not your responsibility to go around and figure how many employees are in which company. Your human resources department or health plan benefits administrator can tell you this. It's just that you need to be aware that if you work for a company with less than 20 or less than 100 employees, your plan may not be classified the way you think it might be.

It is possible that your employer may offer a special plan, not for all employees, but only for those that have Medicare. These special plans are often nothing like the retirement plans specifically designed to work with Medicare. In fact, your employer or union is not allowed to offer a plan that pays Medicare supplement benefits for you (e.g., deductibles or coinsurance). It can offer a plan that pays only for that which is not covered by Medicare (e.g., eyeglasses, hearing aids, dental care, or massage therapy). You should consider such a plan if it's the only one you can get in retirement, or if you have a plan (through your spouse, for instance) that already works with your Medicare.

2.3 Consolidated Omnibus Budget Reconciliation Act (COBRA)

There is a third kind of coverage that is employee-related, which is COBRA coverage. COBRA stands for the Consolidated Omnibus Budget Reconciliation Act. The good thing about COBRA is that it lets you continue with Employer Group Health Plan (EGHP) insurance when you choose to leave work, retire, or some other event occurs relating to your employment (e.g., you get fired or your work hours are reduced so you no longer qualify for your employer's health plan).

If you decide that you want to have this coverage, it's usually called COBRA continuation coverage. You have the right under federal law to keep the coverage you had, but be aware that there are limited time frames on how long you can keep this continuation coverage. Usually, this time frame lasts 18 months. In some cases, it may be extended because of disability or because you get Medicare. Note that divorce, legal separation, death of the covered worker, or loss of dependent child status may also be reasons for receiving this coverage, but as these are not directly related to Medicare, they are not discussed here.

Everyone should be aware that the American Recovery and Reinvestment Act of 2009 provides, temporarily, for both an expanded eligibility for COBRA and a premium reduction to certain qualified individuals on COBRA.

If you were offered Federal COBRA continuation coverage as the result of an involuntary termination of employment anytime beginning September 1, 2008, through the end of 2009, and you either declined to take COBRA coverage at that time or you elected for COBRA and later discontinued it, you may have another opportunity to elect for COBRA coverage and pay a reduced premium. In addition, you may be eligible to pay a reduced premium that is only 35 percent of the premium costs for COBRA for up to nine months. If you have any questions about your situation and how these new rules could apply to you, call the US Department of Labor.

COBRA has a special provision that applies only to retirees — not workers — and only if a retiree's former employer goes bankrupt. If this applies to you, you need to know about this rather unique situation in which you can get COBRA for an extended period of time. If you have retiree coverage and your former employer goes bankrupt, and if there is another company within the same corporate organization that still offers an EGHP to its employees, you will be offered COBRA continuation coverage through that organization's plan. What is so different here (other than this COBRA special provision applying only to retirees) is that you can keep this coverage for as long as you live or as long as that company exists and provides an EGHP. For this reason, this is known as COBRA-for-Life. If this unusual situation occurs, you should get a notice from your former employee about this option. However, if your former employer goes into bankruptcy and you don't hear right away, you should contact the US Department of Labor to see if it can help. These contacts are shown in the COBRA section of the Resources section on the CD.

The law also has a provision that allows the worker's spouse and dependent children, if they were covered under the group plan, to continue their coverage — at least for a while. These dependents can continue their coverage whether or not the individual who was employed does. For example, suppose an employee retires and decides not to continue his or her coverage under COBRA. If that person had a spouse covered under the plan, that spouse can make an independent decision to continue under COBRA or not. This also applies to dependent children who were covered.

Note that you will be responsible for the entire amount of the premium; that is, your old share as well as the company's share. Usually the benefit administrators or insurance company will charge an administrative fee too. There are two good things here, which are that federal law limits the premiums and fees you would pay to no higher than 102 percent of what the company's total premium would be for you (i.e., your share plus the company share). Also, you will get your health insurance at a group rate rather than at an individual rate. This is typically less expensive and provides better coverage. While not required to do so, some companies may help subsidize your premiums. Be aware that your premiums and coverage will change as long as

these changes apply to everyone in the EGHP. Changes typically happen each calendar year.

2.3a COBRA followed by Medicare

If you already have COBRA continuation coverage and you now get entitled to Medicare, your COBRA coverage will end. Note that COBRA has the option to continue, but it probably won't.

Even though your COBRA coverage ends, you will be given the opportunity to apply for a Medigap policy if you sign up for Part B. Therefore, if you want to stay in Original Medicare, you should seriously consider getting a Medigap policy as your Medigap open enrollment period (i.e., guaranteed issue) is limited to six months.

This will only apply if your COBRA plan does not drop you when you get Medicare. If you get Part A only, that would be good because your COBRA will become your secondary insurer. When it ends, and you sign up for Part B, you will also get the opportunity to get a Medigap policy as you are newly entitled to Part B.

If your COBRA plan requires you to sign up for Medicare Part B, you need to make a decision. This is because your opportunity to get a Medigap policy depends on when you are 65 and get Part B. So if you enroll in Part B now, if you don't also sign up for a Medigap policy, you won't be guaranteed issue of a Medigap policy in the future. Your COBRA will probably eventually end, so you'll have to check on how long the plan will let it continue in this situation and at that point you may not be able to get a Medigap policy. Remember, too, that you will be paying the COBRA premiums. The premium for a good Medigap policy will probably be less than your COBRA premium, so if you withdraw from COBRA for a Medigap policy, you will very likely be paying less in premiums and you would no longer have to worry about your COBRA ending.

2.3b Medicare followed by COBRA

You may already have Medicare and begin receiving COBRA continuation coverage later on. This may be because you are 65 or older, but still work; if you retire, leave a company, or are laid off, you can sign up for COBRA continuation coverage. In other words, if you have Medicare and then become eligible for COBRA, you can receive both Medicare and COBRA (but, as mentioned above, you cannot receive both if you become eligible for Medicare after you are already receiving COBRA). Be aware that if you have Medicare Part A, and then get COBRA, and then sign up for Part B or Part D, you get to keep your COBRA because you were already a Medicare beneficiary. If you get COBRA, the effect of this is you have your Medicare and your continuation coverage for a period of time. You can use COBRA as a supplemental policy to your Medicare, but it will eventually end, as typically COBRA coverage ends after 18 months.

You should note that the rules on primary payer and secondary payer for COBRA continuation coverage are different. The size of the former employer is not taken into account, and Medicare is the primary payer. For those entitled to Medicare because of end-stage renal disease, the COBRA is primary payer for the first 30 months of your Medicare entitlement or potential entitlement.

Always remember that your special enrollment period for Part B begins when you lose your Employer Group Heath Plan (EGHP), whether or not you get COBRA. You don't get a special enrollment period when you lose COBRA. Once you sign up for Part B, your Medigap open enrollment period occurs. You have the right to purchase any Medigap policy available in your area, but when your COBRA ends, you will also be given a guaranteed issue right to purchase an A, B, C, F, F-High, K, or L Medigap policy. You need to consider what to do when your EGHP ends. You can join a Medicare Advantage Part C health organization or plan. Or, if you want to stay in Original Medicare, you should get a Medigap policy right away, and forgo COBRA.

For example, suppose you are older than 65 and still working. You got Medicare Part A when you reached 65, but because you had a good EGHP, you decided not to get Part B. You may now want to get Part B, even if you don't need it, because you will not be subject to the premium penalties. If you don't get Part B now, you can only get it in the future during a general enrollment period and you will be subject to the penalties.

If you do sign up for Part B, your Medigap open enrollment period also begins. This is when you have the right to buy a Medigap policy no matter what age you are or what the condition of your health is. This open enrollment period for a Medigap policy will last for six months, and if you don't sign up in that time, you may not get the right to do so later.

Remember, your special enrollment period for Part B occurs when your EGHP ends, not when your COBRA ends. Your Medigap open enrollment period begins when you have Part B and are age 65. Although, you do get a guaranteed issue right when your COBRA ends to buy only certain policies and do it within 63 days. It's probably best to get a Medigap if you don't get a Medicare Advantage managed care health plan.

2.3c Spouses and dependent children

You may also need to understand your dependents' rights under COBRA and how Medicare affects them. As was mentioned in section **2.3a**, if you have COBRA and then get Part B of Medicare, your COBRA ends. However, your spouse's or your dependent children's COBRA does not end. A special rule allows the dependents to keep COBRA even if you don't.

If you, as an employee, got Medicare any-time in the 18 months before you qualified for COBRA and then you get COBRA, your spouse and/or dependent children get COBRA for the normal 18 months plus 18 more months, less the number of months you had Medicare before COBRA. For example, if you are a covered employee that becomes entitled to Medicare 8 months before the date your employment ends, COBRA coverage for your spouse and children would last 28 months (i.e., the 18 normal months, plus 18 bonus months less the 8 months you had Medicare).

2.3d Extension of COBRA rights due to disability

The only reason that COBRA continuation is extended for a worker or employee is if the person is determined by the Social Security Administration (SSA) to be disabled at some point during the first 60 days of continuation coverage. The disability must also continue during the rest of the 18-month period of continuation coverage. If you became disabled (e.g., you had a hunting accident) while you were working and were let go, you got COBRA continuation coverage, and disability existed in the first 60 days of that coverage, and you are still disabled at the end of your 18 months of COBRA coverage, your coverage can be extended; that is, it can be continued for an additional 11 months for a total of 29 months.

COBRA can be a good health insurance bridge if you become disabled. If you become disabled and have to quit work, COBRA will last for the 18 months it normally does, but will be extended for an additional 11 months. This is because when you become disabled, you have to serve a 5-month waiting period to get your Social Security disability, and then receive your disability payment for 24 months before you get your Medicare. This total of 29 months is the length of time you can keep your COBRA. Even

better, your spouse and dependent children will qualify for this extension. At least they can keep this coverage up to the time you get your Medicare, then they are on their own.

As mentioned in section **2.3**, the most you can be charged is 102 percent of the total cost of what the rate is for your employer. Unfortunately, this is not true for the disabled. If you are disabled, you may be charged up to 150 percent during the disability 11-month extension period. Be warned that if you have COBRA and then get disability, you cannot delay telling your plan about your disability so as to keep the lower, regular COBRA premium. You must notify your plan within 60 days after you get your ruling from Social Security that you are disabled.

2.3e Possible post-COBRA conversion rights

You should be aware that you might be able to extend your Employer Group Health Plan (EGHP) coverage even after COBRA ends. While there is no federal requirement for a plan to do so, it may be that your group health plan gives participants whose coverage under the plan terminates the option to convert from group health coverage to an individual policy. If it does, then there is a federal requirement that the plan must give you the same option when your maximum period of COBRA continuation coverage ends. The conversion option must be offered no later than 180 days before your COBRA continuation coverage ends.

Your premium for an individual conversion policy will probably be more than the premium of a group plan, and the conversion policy may provide a lower level of coverage. It is an option that you can explore, and because of the 180-day rule, you'll have time to do so.

Remember that you are not entitled to the conversion option if your COBRA continuation coverage is terminated (e.g., you didn't pay your premiums) before the end of the maximum period for which it was made available.

2.3f State requirements for COBRA

Most states have laws that go beyond federal law and provide for longer periods of coverage or other opportunities, especially pulling firms smaller than 20 employees into COBRA. These are often called mini-COBRA laws for that reason.

Each state's mini-COBRA laws are different, and it's probably best for you to contact your state insurance commissioner to find out what your state's situation is with these laws. If you are at all interested in COBRA but work for a small firm that is not required to have it under federal law, refer to the Resources file on the CD to contact your commissioner's office.

3. Workers' Compensation

The Medicare program has a strong right under federal law to pay only as a secondary payer in Workers' Compensation cases. In addition, if Medicare has made some payments in a Workers' Compensation case, it has a priority right of recovery over any other entity to recover its claim payouts, and it has this right even when a settlement, a judgment, or an award is made. Furthermore, if a settlement, judgment, or award is made which provides for or takes into account the future medical expenses of a worker, Medicare's interest must be considered in Workers' Compensation settlements, even when the worker is not at that time a Medicare beneficiary.

If you are a Medicare beneficiary and you have a work-related injury or illness, you have to tell your employer and file your Workers' Compensation claim. You need to inform the Medicare Coordination of Benefits Contractor about the injury as well. The specific information the contractor will need includes —

- the Medicare beneficiary's name;
- Medicare Health Insurance Claim Number and Social Security Number;
- date of the incident, accident, or illness;
- nature of the injury or illness;
- name and address of the Workers' Compensation insurance carrier;
- name and address of the beneficiary's legal representative, if any; and
- name of the employer.

Once this information is received, the Coordination of Benefits Contractor will update your Medicare record and send you and your representative (if you have one) information about Medicare, Workers' Compensation, the Medicare program's recovery rights. You will also be sent a beneficiary consent to release form to sign and return.

If you had a Workers' Compensation case open prior to Medicare entitlement, questions about this will be on the Initial Enrollment Questionnaire discussed in section 1. You should also know that Medicare does data matching in which it tries to find out if unreported Workers' Compensation payments should be paying for its claims. It's important for you to make sure Medicare knows forthright if you have a Workers' Compensation case open.

3.1 Conditional payment

Your medical claims relating to your Workers' Compensation will go first to the Workers' Compensation organization. It will decide if Workers' Compensation should pay the claims. Workers' Compensation adjudicates your case and pays the bills.

There may be what Medicare terms an extensive delay in getting your Workers' Compensation claim paid if the claim is made by your health-care provider. For example, if your provider of health services files a Workers' Compensation claim, 120 calendar days may elapse without the claim being paid. This typically happens because the Workers' Compensation agency doesn't think it should pay your health care provider, because there is a delay in getting your case set up, or because you are involved in a complicated case. Once the 120 days pass, the provider can file the claim with Medicare in the usual way, and Medicare may make a conditional payment on your claim. However, from this point on, the Medicare program has the right to recover what it paid and you have the obligation to make sure Medicare is repaid.

Medicare makes these conditional payments because your medical expenses may be high and until your case is decided, you probably have only limited means of paying despite your need to continue receiving medical care.

It may be that the Workers' Compensation agency pays some of your claim. This could be if the agency thinks that your illness or injury is only partly related to your Workers' Compensation issue — that is, that it is also partly related to a preexisting condition you had before you took ill on the job. In this case, Medicare may pay on the part of your claim that Workers' Compensation didn't. This payment may be conditional until your case is resolved.

When a settlement, a judgment, or an award is reached, it is important that you or your representative contact the Coordination of Benefits Contractor and tell him or her about it. The contractor will review the information he or she has gathered on what Medicare has paid on your claims and make a decision about how much Medicare is to be reimbursed. The contractor will tell you the amount in what is called a Demand Letter that he or she sends you and that requests that you repay Medicare a stipulated amount.

3.2 Set-aside arrangements

You may reach a settlement with Workers' Compensation that will make sure that you receive money to pay for future medical expenses related to your Workers' Compensation case rather than having the Workers' Compensation agency pay your claims. It is extremely important, if your settlement includes any money to pay for your future medical expenses, that you ask Medicare to look at the proposed settlement to determine if Medicare rights are adequately protected.

The recommended method to protect Medicare's interests is a Workers' Compensation Medicare Set-Aside Arrangement, which allocates a portion of the Workers' Compensation settlement for future medical expenses. The amount set aside is determined on a case-by-case basis and should be reviewed by Medicare when appropriate. This is because once Medicare's determined set-aside amount is spent and accurately reported to Medicare, Medicare will become the primary payer for future Medicare-covered expenses, even if the expenses may be related to the Workers' Compensation injury or illness.

Medicare uses threshold amounts to decide if it needs to review these set-aside agreements. If you are a Medicare beneficiary, the amount is a total settlement (not just medical expenses) of $25,000. If you are not currently a beneficiary but can reasonably expect to be one in 30 months, the threshold amount is ten times this, or $250,000. (This 30-month rule includes those who are age 62 and a half, those who have applied for Social Security disability, and those who have end-stage renal disease but have not yet qualified for Medicare.) It should be emphasized that these are threshold levels that Medicare can change at any time. In every case, Medicare's interests must be accounted for.

Your Workers' Compensation Medicare Set-Aside Arrangement needs to be reviewed by Medicare and should be submitted to the Coordination of Benefits Contractor. In turn, it will send you a letter acknowledging its receipt. This outfit then sends it to a different Medicare contractor: the Workers' Compensation Review Contractor. If you haven't received word of a decision on your proposed Set-Aside Arrangement within 60 days, you can call Medicare to receive a status update.

The actual decision will come from a Center for Medicare & Medicaid Services Regional Office. If you have a question about it, you can contact the Workers' Compensation Coordinator at that office.

Formal appeal rights do not apply to Centers for Medicare & Medicaid Services determinations with regard to Workers' Compensation Medicare Set-Aside Arrangements. However, if you or your representative believes that there is an error in the decision, you can contact the regional office that issued it, indicate what the error might be, and ask for a correction or recalculation. If additional or new evidence is available, you can ask for a re-review of the case by resubmitting it and the new evidence to the Coordination of Benefits Contractor. You always have the right to appeal an individual claim that is denied because of Workers' Compensation.

If you have an amount set aside, use it to pay for your Workers' Compensation related services that Medicare would otherwise cover. You later have to prove to Medicare that you used the money to pay for something it would have paid for. Once this set-aside money is correctly spent, Medicare will begin paying for all services whether or not the services are related to Workers' Compensation. The important message here is you have to keep good records of what you spend and what you spend it on. Remember,

not every legitimate Workers' Compensation medical expense will count, but only Medicare-covered items and services.

4. No-Fault and Liability Insurance

No-fault insurance is accident insurance that is required to pay for the injured party without a determination of who is at fault. It is typically automobile insurance, but it can also be home-owners' insurance or commercial insurance. If a Medicare beneficiary is involved in an accident or a mishap and his or her medical expenses are covered by a no-fault policy, then Medicare will not pay on these types of claims.

Liability insurance, whether it is automobile, homeowners', commercial, medical malpractice, or product liability, is the same as no-fault except there had to be a decision about who was at fault. For example, if a Medicare beneficiary was hospitalized because he or she ate contaminated food, the food processing company would be at fault, and its insurance company (not Medicare) would be responsible for the hospital bill.

If a proper claim is made and denied by the insurance company, Medicare may make a conditional payment on whatever is Medicare-covered. If a proper claim is made and the insurance company does not pay within 120 calendar days, Medicare may also make a conditional payment. Since these payments would be made on your behalf, you would be required to help Medicare recover the payments. If you are involved in a settlement, either a negotiated one or one made through a court judgment of a lawsuit, Medicare will likely recover its payments from the amount you get on settlement.

If even one of your claims is submitted to Medicare and paid, you need to get in touch with the Coordination of Benefits Contractor and let him or her know what the situation is.

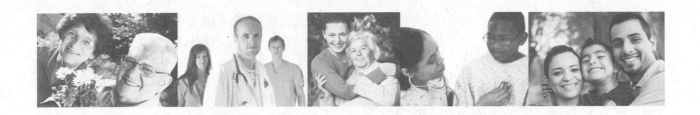

12
Coordinating Medicare with Government-Sponsored Health Programs

The previous chapter discussed how Medicare coordinates with private-sector health insurance programs. This chapter will discuss how Medicare coordinates with government-sponsored health programs.

1. Federal Black Lung Benefits Program

The Federal Black Lung Benefits Program was created by the Federal Coal Mine Health and Safety Act of 1969 to assist coal mine workers who developed black lung disease. This disease is a debilitating and often deadly pulmonary condition. Only former miners are eligible for the medical benefits associated with this program (although certain dependents may be eligible for monthly payments). This program is administered by a component of the US Department of Labor's Employment Security Administration.

The Black Lung Benefits program is a special Workers' Compensation program, and it essentially operates the same with Medicare as any other Workers' Compensation program. If you are a Medicare beneficiary and you also have Federal Black Lung medical benefits, all claims must go to the Federal Black Lung Benefits Program if you seek medical care for a condition related to your lung disease, because Medicare will pay nothing.

For claims not related to the lung condition, Medicare will be the primary payer and you will be responsible for the deductible, coinsurance, or non-covered care. The Black Lung program will pay nothing on unrelated conditions.

It is possible that a Medicare beneficiary has black lung disease, but is covered by a state program, or by a mining company or an insurance carrier. These are also worker compensation programs, and the same general rules apply.

Note in particular that if you have Federal Black Lung Benefits, your prescription coverage through that program is not creditable coverage for purposes of Medicare Part D. This is because the program will only pay for drugs related to black lung disease.

Additional resources to understand this federal program include the Department of Labor's booklet *Black Lung Medical Benefits* (publication CM-6). In the Resources section of the CD, you will find contact information for this program.

2. Veterans Benefits

The Veterans Benefits program is run by the US Department of Veterans Affairs. Veterans benefits are complicated for a number of reasons. There are eight priority groups (many of which have subgroups) of veterans based on each individual's condition, whether their disability or condition is service connected, whether they were a prisoner of war, what their income level is, as well as many other factors that contribute to their eligibility to this benefits program.

Unlike Medicare, the Veterans Benefits program provides most of its care in hospitals and clinics that it runs, but it also uses outside physicians and providers to render care and deliver medical benefits. There is an exception to this general rule. If you are in a hospital and it is not a Veterans hospital, but Veterans Affairs has authorized your care there, and you want to have a particular service that Veterans Benefits does not authorize, the Medicare program will pay for that service if it is covered by the Medicare program. You should make sure the hospital has your Veterans Affairs authorization and your Medicare information.

If you have both Medicare and Veterans Benefits, you will have to decide each time you need medical care whether you want help from Medicare or Veterans Benefits. Basically, if you get your care through Veterans Benefits, Medicare will pay nothing for it. If you decide to go outside the Veterans Benefits system and use your Medicare benefits, Medicare will help pay, but Veterans Benefits won't help at all.

2.1 Coordination of Veterans Benefits with Part B and Part D

As mentioned in the previous section, Veterans Benefits has eight priority groups, from number one (i.e., the highest priority — the richest mix of medical benefits) to number eight (i.e., the lowest priority — it has the least benefits available and the highest co-payments).

If you are in the high priority group, you have much less need for Medicare. If you don't qualify for priority eight, you better sign up for Medicare Part B, Part D, and get a Medigap policy. Note that the VA relaxed its income requirements for priority group eight in 2009. If you applied for it before 2009, you may wish to contact the VA to see if you now qualify.

Veterans Affairs cautions veterans that if they don't enroll for Part B when they are first eligible, having Veterans Benefits will not protect them from having their Part B premiums increased with the normal penalties (i.e., 10 percent for each 12 months they could have signed up but did not). Also note that veterans only have the option of getting Part B when the general enrollment period opens, from January to March of every year, with enrollment effective on July 1 — they do not receive a special enrollment period.

Generally, veterans that do have Veterans Benefits drug coverage do not sign up for Medicare Part D because the Veterans Benefits coverage is quite good and the beneficiary is subject to an $8 co-payment for each month's prescription, with an annual cap of $960 for most priority groups. Some vets are not even required to pay the co-payment. Veterans Benefits drug coverage is considered creditable coverage for Part D purposes, so if a veteran voluntarily decided to sign up for Part D, no premium penalty would apply. Again, the veteran could only apply from November 15 to December 31 of any year, with Part D coverage effective January 1 of the very next year.

In the unusual case that a vet loses his or her Veterans Benefits coverage, the person would be able to take advantage of the Part D special enrollment period everyone gets when they involuntarily lose their creditable coverage. The person has to sign up for a Part D plan within 63 days of the loss of his or her Veterans Benefits. However, Veterans Affairs states that it has never stopped providing medical benefits to those it has already covered.

It is possible that you could lose your Veterans Benefits if you become institutionalized in certain facilities. If you become a patient or inmate in an institution of another government agency (e.g., state veterans' home, state mental institution, jail, or corrections facility), you may not have creditable coverage from Veterans Benefits while in that institution. If you think this might apply to you, Veterans Affairs urges you to contact the institution where you reside, or call the Veterans Affairs Health Benefits Service Center or your local Veterans Affairs medical facility.

Another consideration on whether to get Part B coverage is that you may currently live near a veteran's medical center, but you may eventually move to a place where there is no nearby center. If you have Medicare, you could use it to get care in facilities close to you instead of traveling to a faraway veterans' medical center. Alternatively, you may want to have the ability to choose and have flexibility with your health care, which you can do if you are in both programs. If you didn't like the care you are getting from a veteran's medical center, or the center won't do a certain procedure you think it should, you could choose to have it covered under Medicare.

If you qualify for one of the Medicare Savings Programs that would pay your Part B premium, or if you qualify for the level of Extra Help that would pay all your Part D premium, you should apply for these because you could have premium-free Part B and/or Part D of Medicare as an additional alternative to Veterans Benefits.

If you have a Medigap policy, Veterans Affairs does not bill Medicare for services, but it does bill Medigap insurance companies for services Medicare would cover where those services are given for a non-service connected condition. Even better, if the Medigap insurer pays, this payment is used to offset whatever co-payment you owe Veterans Affairs. Be sure Veterans Affairs knows you have a Medigap policy. For more information on Veterans Benefits, see the contact information included in the Resources section of the CD.

3. Civilian Health and Medical Program of the Department of Veterans Affairs (CHAMPVA)

Veterans Benefits are only available to those who have served in the Armed Forces, but there is a parallel health benefits program called the Civilian Health and Medical Program of the Department of Veterans Affairs (CHAMPVA), which helps pay the cost of health care for veterans' spouses, widows, widowers, and children.

Unlike Veterans Benefits in which veterans get benefits whether or not they have Medicare, CHAMPVA has a very close relationship to Medicare. CHAMPVA almost always requires beneficiaries who are eligible for Medicare Part A to also be enrolled in Medicare Part B to get this benefit. The exception is that some Part A Medicare beneficiaries were grandfathered in some years ago without enrolling in Part B, but anyone now applying for CHAMPVA must apply for Medicare Parts A and B.

If you are eligible for Medicare, you must always enroll in Part B in order to receive CHAMPVA. If you drop your enrollment in Part B, you will be terminated from CHAMPVA. You cannot be reinstated in such circumstances until you apply for Part B in the general enrollment period in the first three months of every year, with entitlement to Part B effective July 1. CHAMPVA will begin on the same date as does Part B, i.e., on July 1.

The eligibility rule applies to those 65 and older, as well as those younger than 65 who are either disabled beneficiaries or end-stage renal disease beneficiaries. End-stage renal disease beneficiaries will be entitled to CHAMPVA for the usual two-month waiting period as long as they elect for Part B to begin with their Medicare entitlement.

If you live outside the US and are eligible for CHAMPVA, you still must be enrolled and paying your premiums for Part B.

3.1 Coordination of CHAMPVA with Part A, Part B, and Part D

If you are entitled to both Medicare and CHAMPVA, you will get an excellent deal when you get a service covered by both programs. In this case, Medicare is the primary payer, and CHAMPVA the secondary payer. You also get pharmacy benefits from CHAMPVA. Further, you will have an annual catastrophic protection limit, so CHAMPVA will cover everything over $3,000 in out-of-pocket covered expenditures in a calendar year. Note that while most families have only one member who is entitled to CHAMPVA, this limit is actually a family limit, so if there is more than one person eligible for CHAMPVA in a family, everything the entitled members spend out-of-pocket counts toward the $3,000.

For simplicity, the following explanation on what is paid for is given as if you have CHAMPVA and Medicare Parts A and B. However, this can be confusing because if you have CHAMPVA and Part B, all of the following are covered by CHAMPVA even if you don't have Medicare Part A. If you don't have Part B, with few exceptions, you won't have CHAMPVA at all.

3.1a CHAMPVA and Part A

If you are hospitalized, CHAMPVA will pay all of your Part A deductible. If you use any of your coinsurance or lifetime reserve days, CHAMPVA will pay all coinsurance amounts up to its allowance (i.e., what CHAMPVA ordinarily pays for a full day of hospital care). You should end up paying nothing out-of-pocket. In the unlikely event you use up all of your Medicare days and it stops paying, CHAMPVA will cover up to 75 percent of its allowance. You will be responsible for 25 percent of any days spent in hospital from that point on.

CHAMPVA will pay all coinsurance amounts for a Skilled Nursing Facility for days 21 to 100 and you should pay nothing. Any days beyond that, which Medicare never pays for, it will cover 75 percent of CHAMPVA's allowance for your covered stay (i.e., what it ordinarily pays for a full day of Skilled Nursing Facility care) and you will be responsible for 25 percent.

CHAMPVA will pay up to its full allowance for your hospice drug co-payments and for respite care, so you should almost always have no liability as these are the only covered items that Medicare does not pay in full.

3.1b CHAMPVA and Part B

Subject to CHAMPVA's own outpatient annual deductible of $50, CHAMPVA will pay, for services covered by Medicare Part B, up to the limit of its full allowance for a service or item, and any Medicare Part B coinsurance or co-payment amounts. These allowances are almost inevitably higher than the Medicare Part B coinsurance or co-payment amounts, so you almost always will end up with no liability, even for the mental health services in which Medicare pays only in part.

The combination of Medicare Part B and CHAMPVA is a very strong one and gives you excellent protection. While you are permitted to purchase both Medigap policies and CHAMPVA supplemental policies, these policies are unnecessary if you have both Medicare Part B and CHAMPVA.

3.1c CHAMPVA and Part D

CHAMPVA has always paid for prescriptions. For prescriptions you get at a pharmacy, CHAMPVA pays 75 percent of the allowable and you pay 25 percent. (The $50 annual outpatient deductible mentioned in section **3.1b** for prescriptions is also included.) It also has a Meds by Mail program, typically used to get prescriptions you take every day or routinely. This program uses the Veterans Affairs formulary to determine if a drug is covered or not. Prescriptions through this program have no coinsurance and no deductible.

With regard to Part D, CHAMPVA is creditable coverage. If you don't sign up for it when you are first eligible, and you decide to do so in a subsequent annual coordinated enrollment period, you will not have a penalty added to your premium. You should also know that if you do sign up for Part D, you will lose your ability to get drugs via the free Meds by Mail program. (This program is available to CHAMPVA beneficiaries only if they have no other prescription drug coverage.) If you decide to enroll in Part D, Medicare will be your primary payer for prescriptions, and CHAMPVA will be your secondary payer. That is, for any prescription, CHAMPVA will pay your Medicare Part D drug

plan co-payment of up to 75 percent of what CHAMPVA would otherwise pay for your drug.

The best advice is to stay with CHAMPVA and not sign up for Part D. This way you can get your routine prescriptions via Meds by Mail and others with only a 25 percent co-payment. The only time you would need to enroll in Part D is if for some reason you cannot get a particular drug you really need in the CHAMPVA formulary but it is in a Part D drug plan's formulary.

One excellent source for additional information is the *CHAMPVA Handbook* which is published by the Department of Veterans Affairs' Health Administration Center.

4. TRICARE For Life (TFL)

TRICARE For Life (TFL) is a major component of the overall health-care system operated by the Department of Defense for both active and retired military service personnel, their family members, and their survivors. Military service personnel include the five branches of the armed services (i.e., Army, Air Force, Coast Guard, Marine Corps, and Navy) and the Commissioned Corps both of the Public Health Service, the Environmental Science Services Administration, and the National Oceanic and Atmospheric Administration. It includes National Guard and Reserve who are in receipt of retired pay. Family members of service personnel include immediate family and former spouses. Note that dependent parents are not eligible.

The discussion in this section will apply to you if you are 65 and retired from the military, or your sponsor is. The term sponsor applies to the person who was in the military and through whom you are entitled to TFL, such as your spouse.

It is likely that your transition to Medicare will be easily managed as the Department of

Defense keeps a database called Defense Enrollment Eligibility Reporting System (DEERS), which tracks all TFL enrollments, and which will know when you are approaching Medicare eligibility. You will receive a notice that you need to apply for Medicare and how to get your DEERS record updated when you get your Medicare eligibility or denial notice from the Social Security Administration. (The Resources section on the CD includes contact information for TFL.)

4.1 Coordination of TRICARE For Life and Part A, Part B, and Part D

If you are either enrolled in Medicare or even eligible for it, you basically have two options on how to receive your care. The most used option is TFL but there is a second, more limited option, known as the US Family Health Plan (discussed in section **4.1c**).

4.1a TRICARE For Life and Part A and Part B

In order to get TRICARE For Life (TFL) you must enroll in Part A and Part B. Medicare becomes your primary payer of health benefits, and TFL becomes secondary. You have the freedom to choose any provider or physician that takes Medicare. The physician or provider will file your claim with Medicare, which will make its payment, and then pass the claim to TFL, which will pay just about any remaining charges. For most of your health care you will be paying the Part B premium every month and that's about it. TFL will even pay your Part A inpatient and Part B annual deductibles. Note that you should never get a Medigap policy if you have TFL because Medigap won't help you much at all.

One thing you should understand about TFL and Medicare is that TFL presumes you will be entitled to Medicare at age 65, and if you are not, you have to prove to TFL that you are not receiving and can't receive Medicare. In effect, at age 65 you will have to file for Medicare

Part A yourself, and you will automatically be filing on your spouse's (or divorced spouse's) account if he or she is age 62 or older.

If you are not entitled to premium-free Part A on any account, you need to make sure that this information gets to TFL. Specifically, TFL wants you to bring your formal Notice of Disapproved Claim, which you will get from your Social Security Administration Regional Office, to a TFL office so that it can enter this in the DEERS and get you an updated identification card. If you are found not to be eligible for premium-free Part A, there will be no change in your TFL benefits.

You should be aware of how Medicare and TFL work when one or the other does not cover a particular service or course of treatment. For services that Medicare covers but TFL doesn't (e.g., chiropractic care), you will be responsible for everything Medicare doesn't pay.

If Medicare doesn't cover something but TFL does, then the rules get a little complicated. TFL has an annual deductible of $100 per individual and $300 per family. Outpatient visits have coinsurance of 20 percent of the negotiated rate of a network provider and 25 percent of the allowable charge for a nonnetwork provider. Preventative, behavioral, and emergency services are the same. For non-covered hospitalization (i.e., the days in excess of your Medicare lifetime reserve days) and Skilled Nursing Facility inpatient care that Medicare does not pay for (i.e., after 100 days of Medicare covered care), you pay up to $250 a day in a network provider and 20 percent of professional charges or $525 per day in a nonnetwork provider and 25 percent of professional charges. The rules for mental health stays are different. The good thing about TFL is that it has catastrophic coverage, so you never have to pay more than $3,000 per year for everyone in a TFL covered family.

4.1b TRICARE For Life and Part D

Medicare and TRICARE For Life (TFL) together are a good combination for health care. With TFL you get a pharmacy benefit and its creditable coverage with regard to Medicare Part D. Ordinarily you do not need to sign up for a Part D plan as your TFL will be as good or better.

You may wish to sign up for Part D if, because of low income and resources, you qualify for Extra Help, and in particular if you can get Part D at no premium to you. If you do not qualify for the Extra Help that pays all of your premium, note that TFL will not pay any of your Part D premium.

The TFL pharmacy benefit is the same as the other TFL programs. You can get your drugs from a Military Treatment Facility via the TFL Mail Order Pharmacy, or at retail network and nonnetwork pharmacies at various costs — it's a flexible program. Note that your out-of-pocket pharmacy costs do count toward the annual catastrophic limit.

4.1c US Family Health Plan

The other option for Medicare beneficiaries is called the US Family Health Plan, which is basically a Health Maintenance Organization (HMO) option. You do not have to have Part B to enroll in this plan, but it helps at lot. This option is geographically restricted and is available only to certain states. In some states it is not offered in all areas of the state.

If you choose this option, you basically get all your care through your HMO, and you can't use other TRICARE For Life (TFL) features such as Military Treatment Facilities, or TFL Prescriptions by Mail. You also have to commit to staying with your HMO for a year.

If you have Part B, you will pay nothing for your care. If you do not have Part B, you will have to pay an annual enrollment fee of $230 (or a max of $460 for a family). You won't have any annual deductible, but you will have to pay $12 for an outpatient or doctor visit (but nothing for preventative services), $30 for an emergency visit, and $25 for an individual outpatient behavior health service. Your hospital inpatient stay will be $11 a day, and the same per day for a Skilled Nursing Facility stay. You also have a $3,000 catastrophic maximum. TFL strongly urges those who can get Part B to do so, even though it is not mandatory.

This option can, depending on the particular HMO you are in, help with other health-related services that are not Medicare-covered, including reduced prices for vision care, hearing aids, and dental work.

5. Federal Employee Health Benefits (FEHB)

If you are a federal employee who had coverage through the Federal Employee Health Benefits (FEHB) for at least five years before retirement, you can continue your benefits into retirement as long as you are willing to keep on paying your share of the premiums.

If you have fewer than five years of service, you must be continuously enrolled since your first opportunity to enroll. Employees can count coverage under TRICARE For Life toward meeting this requirement.

The general rule is to always keep your FEHB. Remember that once you give it up, you can't get it back.

Beginning on the 30th day before you become eligible for Medicare, you may make a change in your FEHB program enrollment from one plan to another or to a different option within your plan. This once-in-a-lifetime opportunity to change plans is yours to take at any time, beginning just before your 65th birthday and with no time limit, but you can do this only once. You can also change plans during the FEHB open season toward the end of every calendar year.

Before you become entitled to Medicare, you should read your FEHB plan's benefits brochure from the perspective of having Medicare as everything changes with Medicare. You want to make sure your FEHB plan is a good fit with Medicare. If it isn't, you may want to change either your plan or your option within a plan. Another good reason to read your FEHB benefits brochure is that sometimes there are quirky rules about how to use your plan, which can change when you get Medicare.

5.1 Federal Employee Health Benefits (FEHB) and Part B

The tough issue for those in Federal Employee Health Benefits (FEHB) who become entitled to Medicare is whether or not to enroll in Part B. There are several facets to this question.

You should know that a FEHB plan cannot require you to take Part B. If you are still working and have had good luck with the plan you have, you may not want Part B at this time, unless you are getting a lot of medical care. You can sign up for Part B at any time if you are still working. When you retire, you can consider getting Part B at that time as you will have the usual special enrollment period of eight months to enroll, and you will not incur any premium penalties.

However, if you do enroll in Part B, with FEHB and Medicare Part A you probably will never get surprised with any high expenses. This is because many FEHB plans will waive your Part B deductibles, coinsurances, and co-payments. (However, even with Part B you still might have to pay excess charges if your plan does not cover them. As a reminder, these are the amounts a nonparticipating doctor or provider can charge above the Medicare approved amount.) You can

get some services at least partly paid for by Medicare if your FEHB plan does not cover them. For example, some plans don't cover all the durable medical equipment Medicare does, some don't cover chiropractic care, and some don't cover home health care that Medicare might, which is basically free to Medicare beneficiaries.

One thing you also want to pay attention to when you read through your plan's brochure when you get Medicare is to see if your FEHB plan gives you a better deal on prescription drugs if you have Medicare Part A and Part B, even though these parts of Medicare don't generally cover prescription drugs. Some plans give lower co-payments for drugs if you have these parts of Medicare, and sometimes a plan will have an option that gives lower drug co-payments to Medicare beneficiaries. Some plans may waive drug deductibles for these beneficiaries so this may or may not give you an incentive to get Part B.

If you are in a Health Maintenance Organization (HMO) under FEHB and you want to continue in it after you get Medicare, you may not need Part B. This is because FEHB HMOs can't require you to get Part B but usually don't give you any additional benefits if you do, so it may not be cost effective for you to get Part B. However, you might want to consider getting it for unusual situations. For example, if you sometimes go out of your HMO network to get doctors or other outpatient services, or if you travel around the country a lot and want to get non-urgent services while you are away from your network.

As some of the FEBH HMO plans are pricey, you should also explore the possibility of suspending your FEHB and getting Part B and then joining a Medicare Advantage Plan. In some parts of the country you can get a really good deal. If you don't like this arrangement, you can, during a FEHB open season, reactivate your FEHB and join a FEHB plan or HMO. (The open season is short, usually from mid-November to mid-December with the changes effective January 1.)

If for some reason your Medicare Advantage managed care plan terminates, or if you move outside its service area, you can immediately enroll in a FEBH plan. Specifically, you must reactivate your FEHB and enroll in a plan in the 31 days before through the 60 days after you lose your Medicare Advantage managed care or health plan.

5.2 Federal Employee Health Benefits (FEHB) and Part D

Federal Employee Health Benefits (FEHB) is creditable coverage for Medicare Part D so you probably will not want to get Part D. However, if you qualify for Extra Help because of low income and resources, particularly if this will pay all of your Part D premium, you should sign up for Extra Help and a good Part D plan.

Another instance in which you might want to get Part D is if you have extremely high drug costs because of the prescription medicines you must take. What you would do in this case is calculate what your out-of-pocket costs are for the drugs. If it is somewhat more than the premiums for a Medicare Part D drug plan available in your state, you may wish to enroll in it if your drugs are in its formulary. Be sure to take into account what your FEHB plan's catastrophic limit is as presumably it will pay all the costs of your drugs from that point on.

5.3 Primary payer rules

If you have Federal Employee Health Benefits (FEHB) because you or your spouse is an active federal employee, and you have Medicare because you are 65 or older or are disabled, FEHB is the primary payer and Medicare is the secondary payer. This is also true if you are a re-employed annuitant and your position is not excluded from FEHB.

If you have FEHB as an annuitant, and you have Medicare because you are 65 or older or disabled, Medicare is the primary payer and FEHB is the secondary payer. This also applies to certain federal judges who officially retired but still work, and former employees getting Workers' Compensation who are certified as unable to return to work. (Their health claims related to Workers' Compensation injuries or illnesses go to Workers' Compensation.)

If you have FEHB and Part B only, Medicare is the primary payer for all Part B services and FEHB is the secondary payer.

If you are entitled to Medicare because of end-stage renal disease, your FEHB will be the primary payer during your first 30 months of eligibility to Medicare and your Medicare the secondary payer. Beginning with the 31st month, this switches and Medicare becomes the primary payer, and FEHB the secondary payer.

5.4 Special rule for retirees who do not have Medicare

While most retired federal employees now have Medicare, some older retirees may have Federal Employee Health Benefits (FEHB) and not Medicare. Interestingly, for most hospital inpatient services and for physician's services (but not for hospital outpatient services), hospitals and doctors cannot charge you more than what Medicare would permit. It's always to your advantage to use a physician that participates in Medicare, even if you do not have it. It is also good to use a hospital or doctor that your FEHB plan recognizes as an in-network or preferred provider. For more information about FEHB, see the Resources section on the CD for contacts.

6. Medicaid

Chapter 1 discussed the general requirements of Medicaid entitlement. If you have few resources and income, you should apply for Medicaid. This is especially true if you have Medicare because one of the general requirements for Medicaid is that you are aged, blind, or disabled. If you have Medicare because of a disability or because you turn age 65, you fulfill these preliminary requirements. Note that Medicaid also recognizes the medically needy, meaning people who spend a large share of their income on medical services. If you are in this position, you should see if your state can help you, especially if nursing home care is involved.

This section deals only with people who are fully entitled to both Medicare and Medicaid programs. This section does not include those who are —

- Qualified Medicare Beneficiaries, where the state Medicaid program pays the beneficiaries' Part B premiums as well as the Medicare deductibles and coinsurances; or

- Special Low-Income Medicare Beneficiaries or Qualified Individuals, where in both cases Medicaid pays the beneficiaries' Part B premiums.

The rule regarding Medicare and Medicaid services is that Medicare is the primary payer, and Medicaid is the secondary payer. Medicaid is always the last payer of medical claims and is sometimes know as the payer of last resort.

Dually entitled beneficiaries of Medicare and Medicaid in effect have to deal with two different and complicated systems of rules and precepts. If by definition they are poor as well as old or disabled, they are likely the least best equipped to deal with these two systems, which don't always work very well in tandem.

If you are dually entitled, services covered by Medicare will have Medicaid pay the deductibles, coinsurances, and co-payments. A physician or provider has to take assignment on the claims for every dually entitled individual. Basically, you should get your medical care paid for, except that some states require you to bear some of the coinsurance or co-payments. You are also eligible to receive services that are not covered by Medicare, but that may be covered by your state's Medicaid program, including long-term care, eyeglasses, hearing aids, and transportation.

You have good coverage with Medicaid so you don't need a Medigap policy. In fact, as discussed in Chapter 11, it is generally illegal for someone to sell you a Medigap policy when you have Medicaid. If you have a Medigap policy and you want to keep it when you get Medicaid, you can suspend your Medigap policy for two years as long as you do so within 90 days of getting Medicaid.

6.1 Medicaid and Part D

Regarding Part D, dually entitled beneficiaries don't have an option; most will automatically be enrolled in a Medicare Part D drug plan. These enrollments are done on a random basis, so it is important that if you are on particular drugs, especially brand-name ones, that you choose a Part D plan that has your drugs in its formulary.

Although you have no option about Part D, you are encouraged to enroll in whichever Part D drug plan you want. You are allowed to switch your Part D plan every month. This is to ensure that you can get the drugs you need. Your cost for drugs will be the same no matter which plan you enroll.

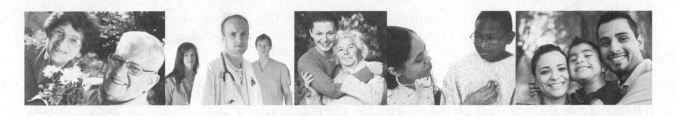

13
Specific Diseases and How Medicare Can Help

This chapter discusses Medicare from the perspective of a few particular diseases, and tries to connect the dots as to what things you should be especially aware of when you or a loved one is faced with a particular disease. It certainly doesn't cover all common diseases, but zeroes in on those where Medicare rules may be a little quirky. Diabetes, heart attacks, and Alzheimer's disease are covered. Because Medicare in particular covers those with end-stage renal disease, and some of the information pertaining to this is very specialized, there is a section about that as well. Details on many of the specific tests and procedures mentioned in this chapter are found in the early chapters of this book.

1. Diabetes

Part D prescription drug plans are required to include coverage for diabetic medications, including insulin. When you select your drug plan, be sure that it covers the specific blood glucose regulator you use. The durable medical equipment benefit covers insulin if it is administered via an infusion pump, which is also covered under the Part B benefit.

Part D law specifies that medical supplies associated with the injection of insulin have to be covered by Part D plans. This means you can get syringes, needles, alcohol swabs, and gauze as part of your prescription drug benefit.

The glycosylated hemoglobin test (HbA1c) is covered for diabetics. Typically your doctor will draw your blood twice a year for this, sometimes more frequently, to determine how well your overall, long-term blood sugar is being controlled. Neither the coinsurance nor the deductible apply to this clinical lab test.

As for the items that you need to monitor your blood sugar level, Medicare Part B does cover the diabetes equipment and supplies you need, whether or not you take insulin. Thus, blood sugar monitors, test strips, lancet devices, and lancets are covered.

Coverage of training is unusual in Medicare, but as diabetics have to take so much personal, daily responsibility for their own care and condition, the program is wise to cover these activities. The two types of training are diabetes self-management training and medical nutrition therapy services. Medicare recommends that nutrition therapy training be taken after the completion of the initial diabetes self-management training.

Medicare usually does not cover eye care, but two extremely important exceptions exist for beneficiaries with diabetes. The first exception is that Medicare covers glaucoma screening as a preventative service for diabetics. Medicare helps pay for a dilated eye examination with an intra-ocular pressure measurement, and either a direct ophthalmoscopic examination or a slit-lamp biomicroscopic examination. The second exception is that Medicare covers diabetic retinopathy screening as a preventative service for diabetics. The screening test is a dilated eye exam.

Medicare typically excludes most foot care, but because of its extreme importance to diabetics, it does help pay for some services here. Diabetic sensory neuropathy, also known as "diabetic peripheral neuropathy," when accompanied with the loss of protective sensations (that is, an inability to feel trauma to the toes or foot), is a serious condition. For those with this condition, Medicare will cover a foot examination every six months (unless you have had covered foot care in the interim). You do not need a referral from a physician to go to a podiatrist for this exam.

Diabetics should remember that while routine foot care is statutorily excluded from Medicare coverage, their particular condition might qualify them for foot care. Where there is already severe loss of sensation in the toes or foot, Medicare may help pay for services of a physician or a podiatrist, even for more common procedures such as removing corns and calluses and clipping nails, where it might be harmful to a diabetic's health for them to do this themselves.

For some diabetics only, Medicare will cover therapeutic shoes, or inserts for your shoes, under limited circumstances. (In the Resources section on the CD, there is contact information to find out more about diabetes and diabetes-related programs.)

2. Heart Attack

This section is certainly not a complete guide to everything Medicare does and does not cover regarding the broad category of heart attacks. However, it does attempt to point out some of the basics. Heart attack victims — whether the attack is real or suspected — will usually be admitted to a hospital as an inpatient, even if only for a brief stay. Medicare will cover this. The following are some of the more frequent heart procedures and tests regarding heart attacks.

Implantable Automatic Defibrillators (also known as Implantable Cardioverter-Defibrillators) are similar to pacemakers; they detect and treat life-threatening tachyarrhythmias. These have been covered by Medicare for some years. The coverage rules are detailed, but include secondary prevention (i.e., you have had a heart attack or arrhythmia, and the device is implanted to help prevent this from happening again) as well as some primary use (i.e., to prevent this condition even though you have not actually had an attack). All primary implants are subject to being involved in data collection for further study by the Medicare program of the medical necessity of this approach and for quality improvement purposes.

Cardiac Pacemakers are programmable, implanted devices that have been covered by Medicare for many years. As could be expected from this long familiarity, Medicare has detailed coverage guides for these, which will be well known by your surgeon. Medicare also has guides indicating how frequently Medicare will pay for the monitoring of these devices. These depend on whether they are the one-chamber or two-chamber types, as well as the overall known reliability of a particular device. Medicare covers Transtelephonic Pacemaker Monitoring as well as Self-Contained Pacemaker Monitors — both digital and audio may also be covered if a physician prescribes them. These durable medical equipment items can be purchased or rented using the usual rules when prescribed by a physician.

Percutaneous Transluminal Angioplasty is done by inserting a balloon catheter into a narrow or occluded blood artery, most frequently a coronary artery, to re-expand it; and is done with or without stents. These are done both as emergency treatments, usually in a hospital; and as elective procedures, often in a cardiac catheter lab. Medicare has long covered this procedure.

Implantation of heart pumps or Ventricular Assist Devices can be covered under certain, specific conditions when used after open-heart surgery as temporary help while awaiting a heart transplant, or as a permanent device to help the heart circulate blood. The Centers for Medicare & Medicaid Services restricts the facilities that can perform this, and is gathering information that it will use to determine whether a facility that does a high volume of these gets better outcomes.

For symptomatic coverage, your physician may order that you have your electrocardiography (EKG) taken while not in the office. This ambulatory monitoring, which involves you wearing a monitor and then using tapes, phone lines, or Internet services to transmit the reading to a physician, a hospital, or an Independent Diagnostic Testing Facility, are covered when medically necessary. Even though equipment is involved, this is not considered a durable medical equipment benefit as the service is a diagnostic package.

Another heart-related ambulatory diagnostic procedure is ambulatory blood pressure monitoring, which Medicare covers if you have a strange symptom, quite descriptively called white coat hypertension (i.e., you see your doctor's white coat and your blood pressure soars in anxiety). This process is similar to EKG ambulatory monitoring.

Heart transplants are covered, but as for all major organ-transplant procedures, only if Medicare specifically approves the hospital to do these procedures. Note that if you do not get your transplant in a Medicare-approved facility, Medicare will not pay for your immunosuppressive drugs. There is no longer any limit for how long Medicare will cover these drugs for a heart transplant or, for that matter, any transplant.

For patients who are waiting for a donor heart to become available for transplant or, for patients who cannot receive transplants, Medicare covers artificial hearts when two criteria are met. One is that the device that is implanted is part of a study that the Food and Drug Administration (FDA) has approved; the other is that certain Center for Medicare & Medicaid Services' clinical research criteria are met. (In the Resources section on the CD, there is contact information to find out more about transplants.)

3. Alzheimer's Disease

Medicare is probably not a very good program for those suffering from Alzheimer's disease, because generally, as the disease advances, a greater proportion of the care needed by the victim becomes nontherapeutic custodial care, which is something Medicare does not cover. Typically costly services such as personal care homes, nursing home custodial care, adult day care in the community, relief care, and home aide services are not paid for by Medicare.

This is not to say that Medicare won't help. Of course it will cover medical services such as some neurodiagnostic testing and medication management, and psychological therapy when provided to patients with Alzheimer's disease, and in some cases will cover a Positive Emission Tomography (PET) scan to diagnose the disease. Although Medicare helps only a percent of those diagnosed with Alzheimer's disease, drugs purchased with the help of Part D help slow the progress of the disease in some victims.

The hospice benefit is apparently not used much for mental conditions with one exception, and that is Alzheimer's disease. In the last few years the medical policy has been revised to clarify coverage of this benefit, but typically it covers only the last stage of the disease, and it's probably best to inquire of a hospice if it believes this would be covered in a particular case.

For mental health in general, you may wish to order the pamphlet *Medicare and Your Mental Health Benefits* (CMS Publication 10184) by contacting Medicare. In the Resources section on the CD, there is contact information to find out more about Alzheimer's disease.

4. End-stage renal disease

Chapter 1 discussed how the treatment of this disease, by preparing for a kidney transplant, getting a kidney transplant, or by beginning dialysis, actually brings entitlement to Medicare for a covered worker, his or her spouse, or his or her dependant child. It also gives the details on when entitlement begins. There is a special provision that if you have Medicare Part A but not Part B when you are diagnosed with this disease, you get a new initial enrollment period to join Part B, and you will pay only the standard premium (adjusted for your income) for Part B. This is extremely important as dialysis is almost always a Part B service. There is a special equity provision so that, if you already have Part B but have been paying a late penalty premium, it will be adjusted back to the standard premium (again, adjusted for your income). Note that none of these special provisions apply to Part D.

4.1 If you have Medicare and then get end-stage renal disease

One of the interesting things about Medicare entitlement is you can actually be dually entitled. Even if you already have Medicare because you are age 65, the Social Security Administration advises that there are four occasions when you will want to file for Medicare based on end-stage renal disease, which include:

- You have Part A but not Part B because you declined it or failed to pay your premiums. You can now get a new individual enrollment period and enroll in Part B at the standard rate, adjusted for income.

- You have Part B, but are paying a premium penalty. Your penalty will be eliminated, and your premium will change to the standard rate, adjusted for income.

- You have Premium Part A. That is, you did not have the required number of work credits (i.e., quarters of coverage), usually 40 credits, to get completely free Part A. It may be, depending on whether you have some quarters and earned them in the period just before you got end-stage renal disease, you will now qualify for premium-free Part A.

- Although this would be a rather remote possibility, you could actually qualify for Medicare earlier than you did as a recently entitled, age 65 or older beneficiary. This would probably entail your getting end-stage renal disease just after you filed for Social Security, or having some issue about the number of work credits you have. If you have recently enrolled in Medicare and gotten the disease, be sure to check with Social Security.

You should be aware that because of the different quarters of coverage requirements for

Social Security payments and end-stage renal disease, it's possible for you to have Medicare and not get Social Security even though you meet the age requirement.

You should also know that if you already have Medicare because you have a disability, and you then develop end-stage renal disease, you should file to get your entitlement based on this disease. There are two general reasons for this. One is that it's possible that you will recover from your disability; if so, your Medicare will eventually stop. If this doesn't happen, getting dually entitled will give you some of the rights discussed above. Specifically, you can sign up for Part B and, if you already have it but are paying a penalty, this penalty will be removed.

Even if you are entitled to Social Security disability but you are in your 24-month long qualifying period for Medicare, or you are scheduled to get your Medicare very soon, you should always file for end-stage renal disease because it may well be possible to establish an earlier effective date for your Medicare. If you are in your five-month waiting period to get your disability payments, you should always file, for the same reason. In this case it is possible for you to get your Medicare before you even get your disability payments.

4.2 A special note on delaying your filing for Medicare

Before you sign up for Medicare based on end-stage renal disease, you need to be aware that it might be in your interest to delay filing. This applies only if you have extremely good coverage under an Employer (or Union) Group Health Plan, which you may have because of current or previous employment. Extremely good coverage means you are subject to either little or no coinsurance or deductible, or you have a very low catastrophic coverage threshold, or both. If your plan has no or very few limitations or caps on services or drugs, you might want to put off filing for Medicare for a time after you get the disease. This is because for the first 30 months of your disease, your Employer Group Health Plan, and not Medicare, will be the primary payer, and it may not make all lot of sense for you to pay Medicare Part B premiums.

The rules on this are very complicated, and they also involve issues such as Medicare payment of immunosuppressive drugs (which you will need if you have a transplant) and the fact that end-stage renal disease beneficiaries have some discretion on when they get Part B.

The best advice is that you should get Medicare as soon as you can unless you fully research the issue and get some good advice about it, because it is complicated. This is because you can file for Part A and reject the Part B. This way you don't have to pay the Part B premiums. However, when you go to get Part B, you can only enroll during the general enrollment period (i.e., January 1 to March 31 of every calendar year). Part B will not begin until July 1 of the year you enroll. You may have a gap in which your Employer Group Health Plan does not pay and Medicare won't either. You will also be subject to the Part B premium penalty, which is 10 percent for every 12 months you could have been enrolled but were not. (The special provision for end-stage renal disease beneficiaries for not having to pay penalties on your Part B premiums applies only if you already have Part A and now get B, or if you are already paying penalties on your Part B.) Because of these factors, the Social Security Administration discourages people from delaying enrollment in Medicare, which is probably quite wise.

If you enroll in Part A and not Part B, there is another bad possibility. You might lose your health insurance (e.g., maybe your company fires you or it goes bankrupt). In this case, you can't get Part B until a general enrollment period begins, which is January through March, and your Part B won't be effective until July 1. In theory there could be a gap of up to 15 months without Part B. This prohibition against giving end-stage renal disease patients a special enrollment period that others are allowed applies to those who are eligible for Medicare because of this disease, and those beneficiaries who have end-stage renal disease even though they have their Medicare because they are older than 65 or disabled.

You do not have to apply and sign up for Medicare when you are first eligible. You can file your application at any time, and elect the month you want to get Part A. (Remember that an application for Part A can be retroactive but the retroactivity cannot go back further than the month you meet other requirements, and it is prospective for three months.) Your filing date for Medicare also creates your opportunity to enroll in Part B using the rules for your individual enrollment period (see Chapter 1). It is possible for you to time your entitlement to Part A and Part B to just when the 30-month coordination period ends (i.e., you would file in any of the three months just before the month your 30-month coordination of benefits period ends). That way your Medicare Part A and Part B can start in that month.

Immunosuppressive drugs are very expensive. If you get a transplant, you will need these drugs. Medicare has a special rule about paying for these drugs. It will cover them under Part B, but only if you have Part A —

- when you had your transplant and Medicare paid for it, or

- at the time of transplant but Medicare did not pay for it because it was the secondary payer and your employer group health plan was the primary payer.

If you take the option of not enrolling in Part A and then you get a transplant without having Part A, Medicare will never pay for these drugs even after you sign up for it. It's not a good idea to delay filing for Medicare if a transplant is an option. Be aware there is some bad information you may come across that says you have to have Part A and Part B when you get the transplant. You do have to have Part A, but you'll have to have Part B to pay for the drugs once your coordination of benefits period ends.

4.3 End-stage renal disease beneficiaries and Medicare Advantage

Chapter 1 mentioned that if you become entitled to Medicare as an end-stage renal disease beneficiary, or if you are already a Medicare beneficiary and then develop this disease, you can't join a Medicare Advantage or managed care plan. However there are exceptions to this rule, and you may want to explore them.

One exception is that if you already have Medicare and are in a Medicare Advantage Plan, and you then develop this disease, you can stay in your plan, or even switch to a plan operated by the same company in the same state. This second provision can help protect you if you move within a state.

If you have end-stage renal disease and are in a Medicare Advantage Plan and it gives up or loses its Medicare contract or reduces its service area so that you are no longer a member, you get a one-time right to join another Medicare Advantage Plan in your area. If your plan leaves, you can switch right away to any other plan that is conducting enrollments. You can wait and join an available plan that is accepting new enrollments at any time.

There are other possibilities for managed care. For one, a Special Needs Plan may be available in your area for those who have end-stage renal disease. These Special Needs Plans are supposed to carefully coordinate your care and are incentivized to report on quality of care, which may be a good approach for you. For another, Medicare, from time to time, has managed care plan "demonstration projects" that take end-stage renal disease beneficiaries. These are temporary arrangements and at any point in time there may one in your area. Probably the best way to find out more about either of these possibilities is to contact the end-stage renal disease network for your state (see the Resources file on the CD for contact information).

You are permitted to join a Medicare Advantage Plan no matter why you are entitled to Medicare, provided you have had a kidney transplant that has restored your kidney function or if you no longer require a regular course of dialysis to maintain life. This is true even if you continue to be entitled to Medicare solely because of end-stage renal disease. (Remember, you'll continue to be entitled for 12 months after your last dialysis treatment or 36 months after your successful kidney transplant.) You'll need a letter from your doctor documenting that you don't need dialysis or that your transplant is working. If you want to join and the plan doesn't seem to know that you can do this, contact the Centers for Medicare & Medicaid Services Regional Office. (See the Resources file on the CD for contact information.)

4.4 Termination of Medicare for end-stage renal disease beneficiaries

Unlike aged beneficiaries, your Medicare coverage can be terminated, although this doesn't happen often. If you get a successful kidney transplant, your Medicare coverage will end on the last day of the 36th month after the month of the transplant. In the unusual case that you no longer need dialysis treatments, your coverage will end on the last day of the 12th month after your last month of dialysis. In other words, you get a full 36 months after your transplant or a full 12 months after your last dialysis of coverage before the termination of your entitlement. Should you have to, during either of these periods, either get a new transplant or begin dialysis, coverage won't end. For example, suppose you had a transplant and things were going well, but 30 months after the transplant you have to go on dialysis. In this instance, your Medicare continues.

If these events happen, the Social Security Administration will notify you that your Medicare entitlement will be ending several months before your actual termination. Its notice will include a "Chronic Renal Disease Medical Evidence Report" (Form CMS-2728). You can submit this form back to Social Security if you do believe your entitlement should not end.

Finally, you should remember that when your entitlement ends 36 months after a successful transplant, Medicare will no longer pay for your immunosuppressive drugs.

4.5 Treatments and options

The following sections discuss the treatments and options available to those people with end-stage renal disease.

4.5a Dialysis

Most people diagnosed with end-stage renal disease will go on dialysis. For many people, they choose to have their dialysis accomplished in an end-stage renal dialysis facility, usually called a dialysis center. These facilities are specially certified by Medicare.

Under Medicare, your dialysis is paid for under a composite rate system. This system wraps up the payment for most of the services you receive into a set fee for each dialysis treatment. These rates vary widely depending on the type of facility, where it is located, the patient's age and health conditions, as well as other factors. Pediatric patients' rates are much higher. Medicare will establish the specific rate for your treatment. Medicare will pay 80 percent and you will pay 20 percent, which is the usual for Part B services. In addition, Medicare rolls your nephrologist's services into a single payment for a month; this is called the monthly capitation payment. It's based on your age and the number of dialysis sessions you have in a month.

There are other costs as well, such as lab tests. While most tests are rolled into the composite rate (whether or not they are actually performed in the facility or sent out to a lab), you may need to have more of these tests that are covered under the composite rate. Some tests that are usually given quarterly (e.g., serum aluminum and serum ferritin) are not part of the composite rate. However, Medicare pays 100 percent of clinical lab tests, so this should not be of concern to you.

Another cost is drugs. Again, many of the drugs you will need are in the composite rate, many drugs are not. You can get an up-to-date list of the drugs from your dialysis center or your network. Unlike clinical lab tests, you will have to pay the Part B 20 percent coinsurance on the drugs.

Regarding dialysis in a facility, Medicare does not cover your transportation to or from your dialysis center. If this is a problem, your facility's social worker may be able to help you. The exception to this is that sometimes ambulance transportation between your home and your dialysis treatment may be covered. It can be covered only if transportation by other means would be harmful to your health. Such indications can include emergency situations (e.g., the patient is in shock), the patient is totally bed confined, or the patient can only be moved by stretcher (e.g., the patient has an unset fracture). Your physician will have to provide a written order for this, and this will have to be renewed every 60 days. Medicare will reimburse you only for getting you to the nearest place you can get dialysis, not necessarily the place you usually go.

Some end-stage renal disease patients elect to go on dialysis at home, and as there are different modalities of home treatments, you and your doctor will have to figure what works best for your situation.

For home dialysis, you will need a trained helper, and Medicare will pay for a family member or friend's training, but it will not pay for a dialysis aide to help you at home.

If you decide to do home dialysis, you will have to choose whether or not you wish to work with a dialysis facility to get all your services, equipment, and supplies, or whether you want to use a durable medical equipment supplier. These are known in Medicare as "Method I" and "Method II," respectively. Once you choose a method, you'll have to live with that method for the rest of that calendar year. While you can choose to go from home dialysis to facility dialysis or vice versa at any time and you may switch the dialysis facility that is supplying your home dialysis, you can't change from Method I to Method II or vice versa except on January 1.

If you go for Method I, Medicare will pay its share of the composite rate and you'll pay 20 percent.

If you choose Method II, you will have to get a durable medical equipment supplier to furnish all your equipment and supplies to you. That single supplier will also have to have an agreement with a dialysis facility to supply you with the services you need to support your home dialysis. These include visits to your home to check on your dialysis, or the equipment or the water supply it uses, or to help in an emergency.

If you choose Method II, your supplier, even if it doesn't participate in Medicare, must take assignment, so the supplier must accept the approved amount that Medicare establishes as the price of the equipment, supplies, and services. (This is an exception to the rule that an enrolled but nonparticipating supplier can charge whatever it wants.) Medicare will pay 80 percent and you will pay 20 percent.

If you go with either method, the facility or the supplier has to get all the equipment to your home and install it in the room in which you will be using it. This includes hooking it up to existing electrical and plumbing supplies, but not rewiring or replumbing your home to accommodate this.

The important consideration in going on Method II is that dialysis equipment is classified as durable medical equipment, which is always rented because of high maintenance needs, so you won't have the purchase option.

You will have time to investigate your options and choose which method you want as you will have to go through training first. The training will be done by a dialysis facility. You make the selection of which method you want to use by having the dialysis facility submit the election form *ESRD Beneficiary Selection (Home Patients Only)* (Form CMS — 382), to its Medicare Administrative Contractor.

Regardless of which Method you choose, on home dialysis your supervising physician (almost always a nephrologist) will be paid based on a set monthly capitation amount, which is a monthly management fee based on your age, and not the number of treatments, as is the case for facility care. Only this set amount for home management is paid, even if during a month you go from facility to home or vice versa.

One other issue regarding home dialysis is the coverage of drugs. These are not an issue with dialysis center patients, as their drugs are given by, or under the supervision of, a physician. To make home dialysis comparable, Medicare law permits Part B to pay for some drugs even when not administered by a physician. More specifically, within the composite rate it will pay for heparin, its antidote, and topical anesthetics. In addition to the composite rate, it will pay for erythropoietin (EPO) therapy for some anemic patients on home dialysis who have to inject these drugs.

Many dialysis patients are capable of travel, but have to be certain of getting their dialysis treatments while traveling. Original Medicare accommodates this as it will pay for treatments no matter where beneficiaries travel in the United States. Medicare Advantage or managed care plans are required to cover dialysis while their enrollees are out of their normal service area. These plans can't require prior authorization of dialysis; but it is best to make payment arrangements between your plan and a facility ahead of time. The problem is trying to line up a facility that has the willingness to take a patient it is not familiar with and that has an open dialysis station for your sessions. If your regular facility is part of a national chain, it may be able to help you locate another chain facility to accommodate you in the place where you will be going. The end-stage renal disease networks (discussed in section 4.6) have extensive contact information and can help with travel information.

4.5b Transplants

Kidney transplants are seen as the preferred treatment of end-stage renal disease. Medicare covers transplants, but only if the procedure is performed in a hospital approved by Medicare.

If a live person donates a kidney, the live donor doesn't get Medicare, but his or her expenses are billed through the Medicare beneficiary to the program. The donor's inpatient hospital stay is fully covered and is not subject to any inpatient deductible or coinsurance. If your donor should suffer any complications for the transplant, the complications are covered. Any Part B services are also approved at the going Medicare rate and Medicare pays its share (usually 80 percent) and the beneficiary (not the donor) pays 20 percent. There is never a Part B deductible for the services given to the donor.

In regard to the blood deductible, if a live donor gives blood for a transplant (this is sometimes done to assist the acceptance of the transplanted kidney in the recipient's body), this blood is considered replacement and does count toward your three-pint deductible.

There is a special exception to the general rule that dental services are not covered by Medicare. If you are going to have a kidney transplant, a dental exam made to determine if your teeth or gums might cause an infection if the transplant were to go forward is covered by Part A if done by a dentist on the hospital's staff, or Part B if done by a physician.

The recipient and the potential donor will have to have exams and tests performed to ensure that both of you are healthy enough for the transplant and that you are compatible with the donor. These tests are covered under Part A, and are covered even if done in a hospital that is not an official transplant hospital. The physician services are covered under Part A, but you will not see a separate charge for these as they are billed as a "kidney acquisition charge" by the transplant hospital to Medicare. Because Medicare deems that preadmission tests are done as part of the transplant, these tests will be covered even when the beneficiary may not have been Medicare eligible at the time the tests were done either to the beneficiary or donor. Also, any necessary kidney registry fee is covered under Part A.

4.6 End-stage renal disease networks

The basic purpose of end-stage renal disease networks is to monitor and improve the quality of care end-stage renal disease patients receive. Medicare law requires anyone diagnosed with this disease who gets a transplant or starts dialysis to be entered into a database that the government uses to help register people for transplants, maintain quality in dialysis facilities, collect data for research, and to help them enroll in Medicare if they are eligible. This information is sent from transplant hospitals and dialysis facilities to these networks and on to a national database.

Another function of the end-stage renal disease networks is to educate and inform patients about the disease, to encourage them to take an active role in maintaining their health, to promote kidney transplants and the use of home dialysis, and to ensure patients adjusting to work issues know about available vocational rehabilitation programs. When you are first registered, your network will learn about you and will send you a packet of information, as well as the network's contact information. Your network can be a very helpful source of information to you, particularly because it is located in your area of the country and it is knowledgeable about conditions there. (The contact information for end-stage renal disease networks is included in the Resources file on the CD.)

One right you have when being treated for end-stage renal disease is to avail yourself of a formal grievance process that is run by these networks. If you are unable to resolve issues with your provider or practitioner, you can file a complaint or a grievance with your network.

When you contact your network with your concern, it is supposed to discuss the issue with you, and you have to be given the option of deciding if it's a complaint or a grievance. The difference is that a complaint will result in a fairly informal and quicker attempt to work on the issue and resolve it, while the grievance process is a formal process.

You should be aware that you can file a complaint or grievance anonymously, or you can file a complaint or grievance with the proviso that your name or identity not be disclosed in pursuing it. This may lower the chance of getting the issue resolved. You can download from the Medicare website a brochure called *Filing a Complaint Concerning Dialysis or Kidney Transplant Care* (CMS Publication No. 11315) for more information.

If you do file a grievance, the network is supposed to resolve the issue in 90 days; however, this is not a hard and fast deadline. If the network proceeds, it will send you a letter acknowledging your grievance and ask for your consent to use your name in pursuing it (you don't have to agree to this); this letter will include the name of a contact person on the network staff whom you can call to discuss the matter or find out what progress is being made. It will thoroughly review the situation and try to come up with a resolution. Because this is a formal process, once the network comes to a conclusion, it is required to inform the provider or facility in writing of its initial conclusion, and allow the provider or facility time to formally respond with its views.

The final response must be in writing. The network may require a facility to go on an "improvement plan" to fix the situation. The letter will also tell you what you can do if you don't believe the formal response was appropriate. This includes contacting the Centers for Medicare & Medicaid Services' Regional Office as your next step. However, at this point your formal grievance rights have been exhausted.

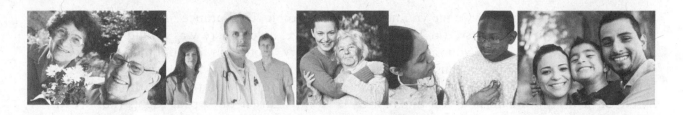

14
Medicare Appeals

Appeals are requests you make to Medicare in an attempt to get it to pay for claims for health services in which it has denied payment. You may also appeal to Medicare if you want to stay in the hospital when it wants to discharge you, or to get care from your Medicare Advantage Plan that it doesn't want to give you. This may be the most critical section in this book — one of the best ways to get Medicare to work for you is through the appeals process.

When the Medicare program makes a decision that is adverse on your claim or service, it almost always has to send you a written notice about what it decided. For example, when it denies a claim for a medical service you received, or it tells you it won't pay for you to stay in the hospital any longer. The notice has to tell you how to appeal the decision. You can follow the process on a step-by-step basis based on the paperwork that is sent to you.

This chapter tries to give you an understanding of how the whole process works, and provide you with some guidance on how to make it work for you as you go through its various steps or levels. On the CD in the file Appeals Steps you will find charts that are useful for quick reference when you have questions about the steps.

1. Some Helpful Guidelines for Medicare Appeals

The Medicare appeals process has steps that you must follow sequentially. Be aware that each step of the appeals process has strict deadlines for you to follow in filing the next level of appeal. Some deadlines are as short as 60 days, while others are as long as 180 days.

You should also be aware that it is always possible to overcome these deadlines for "good cause." For example, you may have been recovering from a long hospitalization for a stroke and you missed a deadline on a particular appeal. Go ahead and file the appeal, and ask that "good cause" be found to extend the deadline. Specify in detail why you think you deserve this extension.

1.1 Amount in controversy

At the higher levels of appeals you have to meet a relevancy test in terms of a dollar amount to file for an appeal. For example, to get a hearing before an Administrative Law Judge you need at least $130 to be "in controversy" (in 2010). This is merely to say that to accept your appeal, a specific, minimum dollar amount must be in question. These amounts usually escalate each year based on a health-care related consumer price index. Also, note that you are permitted to combine claims to meet these amounts.

1.2 Federal rules govern

Remember that because Medicare is basically a federal program you can't use state or local courts or procedures to change the result or ask for relief on a claim.

1.3 Forms

There are specific forms to file for each step in the appeals process. It makes good sense to use them because, if you do, you will send in all the required information for each step. To get these forms, you can call Medicare, or go on the Medicare website; a link to this is included in the Resources file on the CD.

1.4 Other entities appealing

You may file an appeal on any claim that involves you, but so can, in most cases, the facility, provider, physician, or supplier that furnished the service to you, and they can appeal on behalf of your claim whether or not you do. Most appeals are filed by these entities because they are more familiar with the appeals process than individual beneficiaries. If one of these entities appeals, you will become a party to the appeal. In the rather unusual instance in which the entity cannot appeal, you can transfer or assign your appeal rights to one of these entities. They will be the ones to ask you to do this, and it will be to your advantage to do so.

If you transfer or assign your appeal rights, the transferee has to to waive the collection of any amount due from you except for the applicable coinsurance or deductible for the service, unless there was a valid Advanced Beneficiary Notice indicating that the service or item might not be covered by Medicare. This remains true even if they lose the appeal. Use the form Transfer of Appeal Rights (Form CMS — 20031) to assign appeal rights.

1.5 Representation

You also have the right to appoint a representative to carry on your appeal. This may be a family member or friend, or possibly one of the health service entities that is not a party to your appeal, or an attorney, or Medicare advocate. Use the form Appointment of a Representative (Form CMS — 1696) to do this.

Sources for help with representation include State Health Insurance Assistance Program (SHIP) staff and volunteers (the state-by-state toll-free numbers are in the Resources section on the CD), legal aid groups, state and local bar associations, elder law projects, Medicare advocacy or rights organizations, and law school internship programs.

1.6 Escalation

At some of the advanced appeals steps you are given the option of "escalating" the appeal if you don't get a decision in a given time frame. That is, if you want to, you can move your case up to the next level. You don't always have to be notified when the given time frame is expiring so you'll have to keep track yourself. If you ask for this, the entity involved can take five extra days to finish up the case and render a final decision.

2. Original Medicare Appeals

With some exceptions, all Original Medicare decisions with appeals rights are after-the-fact. This is to say that you received a medical service, a claim was submitted, and the claim was denied. By denied it usually means that nothing was paid on the claim by Medicare; however, it may also mean that the service was partly paid for, but at a level or amount lower than was submitted or claimed. These can be appealed as well as a full denial.

The first time you will get news that a claim has not been paid may be with your periodic Medicare Summary Notice, which will also tell you how to appeal.

2.1 Resubmittals

It might not be necessary at this point to appeal if your Medicare Summary Notice shows your Medicare Administrative Contractor denied a claim your provider or doctor submitted because of a simple error (e.g., maybe your provider mixed up your Medicare number). You can usually get these resolved by having your provider or doctor resubmit your claim with the appropriate corrections.

2.2 Redeterminations

A redetermination is your first step in the appeals process. Your Medicare Summary Notice will tell you exactly how to make this appeal. You'll get this notice in the mail about every three months from the Medicare Administrative Contractor which processes your claims; it tells you which were approved and/or denied. The Medicare Administrative Contractor that originally processed your claim will do the redetermination, and you must make your request to it. You must make your request within 120 calendar days of the date of your Medicare Summary Notice.

Requests for redeterminations must be made in writing; however, nothing formal has to be filed. You can write your request on the Medicare Summary Notice you received and mail it back to the address given on your notice. This is a very efficient way to ask for your redetermination. You must clearly indicate which service or services you want redetermined, your reasons for this, and you must sign the request. Make a copy of it before you mail it. Or you can always use the Medicare Redetermination Request (Form CMS — 20027). You may want to get a statement or letter from your doctor or health-care provider and attach it to your request. If you file a statement or other document, be sure to copy it.

You can even initiate this process by phone. The Medicare Administrative Contractor will complete a request for redetermination form and send it to you for your signature so that your request will be in writing.

Once the Medicare Administrative Contractor receives your redetermination request, it must mail you an acknowledgment. Note that it has 60 calendar days to process your redetermination request from the date it was received.

If its redetermination decision is not fully in your favor, the contractor will send you a somewhat detailed letter telling you why it was not in your favor, and how to appeal.

2.3 Reconsiderations

If you did not like the redetermination decision, you may proceed to the next appeals step, which is the reconsideration. Follow the notice you get about your redetermination when you file for this. Note that you must file your request in writing, and you have 180 days from the date on your redetermination notice to file for this. You should use the Medicare Reconsideration Request form (Form CMS — 20033).

While it is not required of you, the beneficiary, it is a good idea at this step to file everything you can that supports you. Be sure to get physician reports, discharge notes, whatever documentation you can that will support your request, and submit them.

All reconsiderations are made by an organization different from the Medicare Administrative Contractor who made the redetermination decision. These organizations are called Qualified Independent Contractors. Your redetermination notice will tell you which one to send it to, or you can call Medicare. The contact information is also included in the Resources section on the CD.

These contractors are supposed to conduct a completely new, on-the-record review of all the material from the redetermination case, anything new that is submitted and anything they gather independently. The contractors must respond to your reconsideration request in 60 days. However, if you submitted more evidence after your initial request, they get an extension of 14 days for each new submission.

The contractor's response must be the decision itself; however, if a decision can't be made within the 60-day deadline, they must send you an escalation notice. The notice will indicate that you have the option of filing for the next level of appeal and it will tell you how to do so.

If the Qualified Independent Contractor does make a decision, you will get a very detailed notice of the decision, its rationale, and what you can do next. This notice will also give you a complete explanation of how you can go to the next appeals level. It will also tell you how you can find out more about the applicable laws and regulations that apply in your case.

2.4 Administrative Law Judge hearings

Your next step is a hearing before an Administrative Law Judge, known as a Medicare Hearing. The notice you get about your reconsideration will tell you how to file for this.

Note that you must file your request in writing, and that you have 60 calendar days after you receive your reconsideration notice to do so. At this step, the "amount in controversy" requirements begin, so be aware that at least $130 (in 2010) must be in dispute. File the Request for Medicare Hearing by an Administrative Law Judge (Form CMS — 20034 A/B) for this step. Your reconsideration letter will tell you where to mail it.

If you do not indicate that you have a representative, the Office of Medicare Hearings and Appeals is supposed to supply you with a list of representatives that may be able to help you. This hearing step is a more complicated process than the two previous steps, so you should contact a potential representative to see if he or she can assist you.

The Administrative Law Judge will schedule the hearing and then, at least calendar 20 days before it is to take place, send out a formal hearing notice. This notice will set the mode (e.g., videoconferencing, telephone conference call, or in-person hearing), date, time, and place, and will also set out the specific issues that will be decided. You should read this notice carefully and respond to any concerns quickly and in writing.

Unless you ask for an on-the-record decision, you'll get a chance to explain your case in a hearing. While these hearings are non-adversarial in nature, they have many similarities to a court proceeding. You may testify yourself and you may bring others to testify. You have the option to be represented by an attorney or other person (all at your own expense). If you have a complex medical problem causing a coverage issue or a medical necessity issue, you should always try to get your medical professional to accompany you to the hearing or at least to submit a written statement. You may question other witnesses, and examine all the evidence presented by others and even object to the inclusion of any particular piece of evidence in the record.

Once the hearing has been completed, the judge will write the decision and send it to you, and usually also to all those who were involved. The judge's decision will give finding of facts, conclusion of law, the specific reasons for the judge's decision, and will summarize the evidence used in making the decision. You will be told how to obtain more information about the decision, and how you can appeal it to the next step. These hearings are recorded, and you can get a copy of the tape if you appeal to the next level.

You can request an escalation of your case if the Administrative Law Judge hasn't made a decision in the required 90 days.

2.5 Medicare Appeals Council reviews

The Medicare Appeals Council is part of the US Department of Health & Human Services' Departmental Appeals Board (DAB). It functions similar to an appeals court to the individual Medicare Administrative Law Judges. Again, when you get your notice of an Administrative Law Judge decision it will tell you how you can file for your review. Basically, it will instruct you to file a DAB Request for Review Form (Form DAB — 101).

You must file your request for review within 60 days of your Administrative Law Judge decision. Note that no amount in controversy requirement applies here.

You should include any supporting evidence or documentation, if it is not already part of the case record; however, the Council does not necessarily have to consider it. Typically the Council does not have an appellant appear before it, although you have the right to ask for this. It also has the authority to compel limited discovery and issue subpoenas. It has 90 calendar days to make its decision.

If it has not made its decision within the appropriate time frame (i.e., 90 days when you file for a review, or 180 when you escalate), you may ask in writing that it escalate your appeal.

2.6 US Federal District Court suits

Your final appeal step is to go into the federal court system, and file a civil action against the Secretary of the US Department of Health & Human Services in a federal district court. You have 60 calendar days from the day you receive the notice of the decision by the Medicare Appeals Council and the amount in controversy has to be at least $1,260 (in 2010).

Unlike the other appeals steps, you do need an attorney who has been accepted to practice in such a court. You may be able to find an organization to assist you because the organization may think a precedent needs to be set that a certain surgical procedure or medical device should be covered by the Medicare program.

2.7 Your right to receive notice of and to appeal the termination of four specific services

You have a right to appeal when your health care provider tells you that services you are receiving in four specific provider settings will be ended. This applies when you are receiving inpatient hospital care, Skilled Nursing Facility care, Home Health Agency services, or Comprehensive Outpatient Rehabilitation Facility services. Note that this right generally includes the requirement that your provider notify you that the services will be ending and how to contest this.

You should also understand the reasoning behind this right. The Medicare program, to control its burgeoning costs, has generally shifted paying for care from a "cost" basis to an "incident" basis. For example, your hospital will be paid for your inpatient stay not based on how long you are there but based on your age, diagnosis, or what surgery you had. This special appeal right was instituted to give you some counterbalance to these providers' strong financial incentive to discharge you as soon as possible.

The good thing about this right is that your appeal is made to an outside organization, in this case, the Quality Improvement Organization that serves the state in which your provider is located so you get a completely independent review. You can't be discharged or have services ended until the organization makes its ruling. You don't have to do this in writing, just make a call.

2.7a Inpatient hospital care

Whenever you go into a hospital as an inpatient, you will be given a two-page document called "An Important Message about Your Medicare Rights." It will inform you that when you are told that the hospital is about to discharge you, you have the right to appeal that decision.

When the hospital sees that you are getting ready to be discharged, it will give you another copy of the document. It should do so at least two days before your discharge, but it must give it to you at least four hours prior to discharge. To appeal your discharge you call the toll-free number of the Quality Improvement Organization that is shown on the document. You can call at any time, day or night, seven days a week. Even if you just leave a message, your appeal has begun. The hospital may not discharge you until the Quality Improvement Organization makes a decision about your discharge. For you not to incur any liability for your stay, you must call the Quality Improvement Organization *before* you are discharged.

Once you have called the Quality Improvement Organization, it then notifies the hospital that you have appealed. The hospital has to give you a "Detailed Notice of Non-Coverage," which tells you why the hospital thinks you should be discharged. This is not a discharge order; once you have appealed, only the Quality Improvement Organization can decide whether you should be discharged.

The Quality Improvement Organization will solicit the views of the hospital, your physician, and you. After gathering your medical records, it will make a ruling and call you with its decision. It may possibly prolong your stay by requiring the hospital to set a new discharge date. Or it may decide that your discharge is appropriate; if this happens, you become liable for your stay beginning at 12 noon on the very next day after it calls you with the decision.

If the Quality Improvement Organization decides that you should be discharged, and you are willing to personally risk the liability of paying for additional hospital care, you can make arrangements with the hospital to stay. (You may have to give the hospital a substantial deposit.) In this case, you can appeal to the Quality Improvement Organization's decision to the Qualified Independent Contractor. Information on how to do so will be in the written notice you get.

This appeal is known as an expedited reconsideration request, also knows as a "Fast Track Reconsideration — 72-Hour Turnaround Request," which you make while still an inpatient. You can make your request by phone. The Qualified Independent Contractor has to make a ruling within 72 hours of your request. It will notify you by phone, and will tell you what your liability is in your situation and, if the decision is not wholly in your favor, how you can appeal.

It is possible that you can be given other notices that affect Medicare coverage of your hospital stay. It may be that you are being considered for admission for what might be a covered stay and the hospital decided that your stay won't be covered. In these cases the hospital will issue you a "Preadmission/Admission Hospital-Issued Notice of Non-Coverage." It will have information in it on how you can appeal it.

2.7b Skilled Nursing Facilities, Home Health Agencies, Comprehensive Outpatient Rehabilitation Facilities, and hospices

If you are an inpatient in a Skilled Nursing Facility (SNF), or you are receiving a course of treatment from a Home Health Agency, a Comprehensive Outpatient Rehabilitation Facility (CORF), or a hospice, your provider cannot discharge you or discontinue your services until you have had the opportunity to appeal. This appeal is made to the Quality Improvement Organization that serves the state in which the services are being given. You don't have to do anything in writing; just place a call. This special right does not apply when the provider changes the frequency of services (e.g., when a Home Health Agency reduces the number of visits from three a week to two) or when the kind of services change (e.g., a CORF discontinues your physical therapy but continues with your speech therapy).

In these cases you will always get a notice from the health care provider that is treating you. These are called a "Notice of Medicare Provider Non-Coverage." You must get your written notice no later than two calendar days before your discharge or the discontinuation of your services, but in some cases you will get it earlier than this. The notice will specify which day the care is ending, when your financial liability begins, and how you can appeal this. It will not go into much detail. You have until noon on the day after the day you receive this notice to appeal to the Quality Improvement Organization.

Once you have contacted the Quality Improvement Organization, your provider will then have to give you a more in-depth rationale for your discharge or the discontinuation of your services. This notice is called a "Detailed Explanation of Non-Coverage." The Quality Improvement Organization will use it, and whatever other medical records it obtains, to make its decision as to whether your care should be extended or not. What's in your favor in these appeals is that the burden of proof is on your provider to demonstrate that the termination of coverage is the correct decision.

If the decision reaffirms your discharge or discontinuation, you have to decide if you will go along with it. If you decide you need more care, you'll be on your own. You can arrange for it, but you will have to either pay it out-of-pocket or hope, that by using the Fast Track Reconsideration — 72 Hour Turnaround Request process for appealing (as outlined in section 2.7a) that you can get a ruling in your favor and require that Medicare pay for it.

2.8 Appeals of local and national coverage determinations

There is a special appeal right open to all Medicare beneficiaries who believe that they will have payment denied for a service they have not yet received, if the denial will be one based on a local or national coverage determination; or if they have already received the service and had their claim denied based on one of these determinations.

Medicare Administrative Contractors are responsible for making coverage policies for any number of reasons (e.g., to deal with issues involving a new medical procedure). These policies are called Local Coverage Determinations, and they apply only in that contractor's jurisdiction. The federal Centers for Medicare & Medicaid Services has a parallel responsibility, but its policies are known as National Coverage Determinations as they apply throughout the nation.

In most cases these appeals are not made directly by the beneficiary but by the physician or provider from whom the beneficiary wants to get the service. This is because a coverage determination tends to affect all the physicians and providers who wish to give the particular service addressed in the determination, and they are concerned not just with the care the beneficiary receives but what will be covered for all their Medicare patients.

There is no specific form on which to make this appeal. You can simply write a letter to the US Department of Health & Human Services' Departmental Appeals Board (DAB). In the letter, include your name, address, phone number, email address, and Medicare number. State the title of the national or local coverage determination that is being challenged, and the name of the Medicare Administrative Contractor that issued it, if it is a local determination. For the substance of the appeal, explain the specific provision or part of the coverage determination that affects you, what item or service is needed, why the coverage determination is unreasonable, and why the appeal request is being made. The letter must include a written statement from the doctor treating you that states that the item or service is or was needed. Your deadline in which to file is within six months of the date of the physician's statement, or within 120 days of the claim denial notice, if you have received the service.

If you are appealing a local coverage determination, your appeal will be assigned to an Administrative Law Judge. If you are appealing a national coverage determination, the DAB itself will review the determination and make the decision.

3. Medicare Managed Care Rights

With Medicare Advantage or managed care, you have some very special and powerful rights; indeed more rights than in Original Medicare. Everything mentioned earlier about your rights as a Medicare beneficiary is magnified in the managed care setting. This is because once you have joined a managed care plan, you are often dependent on that organization to arrange for and provide your care, and you expect to get all the services you need, as well as high quality services.

You have four extensive sets of rights under Medicare managed care:

- Right to a determination: The right to get a decision from your plan on whether it will cover or continue a service or course of treatment. If your condition requires, you have the right to have this decided quickly.

- Appeal rights: The right to appeal any decision by your plan on what services you get, or how much you have to pay for the services.

- Right to file a grievance: The right to formally complain about virtually any aspect of your relationship with your plan.

- Right to express dissatisfaction about the quality of care you receive: These complaints are handled in such a special way that they constitute a special right.

These rights are not mutually exclusive. It's entirely possible for one event or incident that dissatisfies you to trigger more than one of these rights.

You also have some other rights. One is that you have the right to appeal when your plan tells you that services you are receiving in four very specific provider settings will be ended. This is the same right discussed in section 2.7, except that you may get a notice from your plan instead of the provider; these notices will tell you how to appeal. The other is that there is a special appeal right open to beneficiaries who either cannot get a medical service authorized or approved by their plan, or who have had payment denied for a service, if the denial is based on a local or national coverage determination. Again, this works the same way as discussed in section **2.8**.

You also have the right, when you are filing an appeal, to get a copy of all your medical and other information concerning your appeal. Your plan is permitted to charge you a reasonable fee to copy your file and mail it to you. If your appeal goes to the Part C Qualified Independent Contractor, you also have the right to request your file from it.

3.1 Right to a determination

You have a right to receive a determination about your request to your plan for care or for payment. You, in effect, have two completely different sets of rights here. One right comes into play when you have not actually received a medical service that you want to get. The other right concerns having your plan pay for a service you have already received. The following two sections discuss these rights separately as what you need to do to exercise each differs considerably, at least up to a certain point. The key to understanding here is that you deserve a response to your request for care or for payment, and your plan's decision begins the appeals process.

3.1a Your right to a decision to receive care

In Medicare managed care, you always have the right to ask for a medical service or item. You will either get what you ask for, or you will get an understandable and well-reasoned negative response to your request from your plan. For example, if your cardiologist advises you that you need angioplasty, but your plan wants to continue to treat you with prescription medicine, you will not be covered for angioplasty.

You can also ask that a treatment that you are getting be continued at your current level. For example, your plan tells you that you will now be going to your physical therapist only once a week, but you think you should continue your three-day-a-week schedule. Another example is that your current treatment be intensified (e.g., your oncologist wants to increase your chemotherapy sessions from one to two a week, but your plan believes that one is sufficient). Or your established course of treatment should not be stopped (e.g., you are authorized to go to your urologist for a monthly test for recurrence of your prostate cancer, but your plan says this is no longer medically necessary). In any of these examples, your plan must give you a written notice if you request one. If it doesn't, use these guides to get one because you can then appeal.

Typically your first indication that your plan won't give you what you want is an informal "no." If you disagree, and you haven't gotten a formal, written determination, you need to ask for one. Your request should be in writing, because this will give you the documentation you need if your plan fails to respond, or does not do so in a timely manner. Basically these are two approaches you can take to get your decision — the standard time approach or the fast track, expedited approach.

The "standard time" requests for care basically have a 14-day turnaround time. You should be clearly advised by your plan on how to request a decision on your care. (Technically, these are known as "Organizational Decisions".) Your "Evidence of Coverage" booklet or letter from your plan will specifically tell you how to ask for your formal decision. Again, you are strongly advised to always file these in writing. To speed things up, it's fine to call them in, but follow up with a letter or fax — something in writing.

Your request should specifically state just what service or treatment you want to receive, want increased in intensity or duration, or don't want reduced or stopped. Cite your reasons. If at all possible, a supporting statement from your physician or health-care provider should accompany your request. (Your plan may permit these to be called in.)

Your plan has 14 calendar days to respond to you (and it is supposed to do so in less time if your medical condition requires it), although it can extend this in some circumstances.

At any rate, your plan must deliver its written decision to you, and if its decision is not wholly favorable to you, it must include a short document called a "Notice of Denial of Medical Coverage." This must be clear and specific to your situation, and it must tell you of your further appeal rights. If you do not get a "Notice of Denial of Medical Coverage," you have the right to appeal this decision (which is why you should always file in writing and keep the deadlines in mind). Remember that you can appeal if your plan gives you an adverse notice or if you do not get one at all.

"Expedited" requests for care basically have a 72-hour turnaround time. It may be that you, your physician, or your family believes that you have an urgent need for a service or procedure (e.g., a CAT scan). You have the right to ask your plan for a fast track or expedited decision in this case. If you do ask, your plan will make two decisions — one is whether the decision should be expedited, and the other is the decision itself. Note that any physician, not just yours, can also make this request for care.

Your request should have the same information as a standard one. The best way to justify and expedite a request is to get a statement from any physician that supports your request by indicating that your life, your health, or your ability to regain maximum function would be seriously jeopardized by having to wait for a standard time decision. If you submit such a statement, your plan has no choice but to expedite your decision.

In effect, your plan has 72 hours to make its decision and to notify you of it (exceptions sometimes apply). If, within that time frame, it says it will not expedite the decision, but will go with the regular 14-day standard track to make its decision, you can grieve this aspect of its decision. Its notice not to expedite must clearly inform you of this and tell you what your grievance rights are.

At any rate, you will have the actual decision in the 72-hour or 14-day period. If the plan's decision is not wholly favorable to you, your plan must, within an additional three days, deliver to you a "Notice of Denial of Medical Coverage," which will tell you of your appeal rights. If you do not get this notice, you have the right to appeal this lack of a decision.

3.1b Appeal rights

Your "Notice of Denial of Medical Coverage" will tell you what your specific appeal rights are and how to exercise them with your plan. This first appeals step is called a reconsideration. As with your right to a determination, these are two appeal approaches you can take — the standard time or the fast track, expedited appeal. Each topic is discussed separately below, but all reconsiderations have the following in common.

You can choose either standard time or fast track regardless of which track you used to get your determination. For example, if you asked for a standard time determination, but now your condition has worsened and you need a fast decision, ask for an expedited reconsideration. In other words, let your condition decide, not what you did before. The most important safeguard is that if your plan does not now decide your appeal wholly in your favor, it must send your appeal to an organization outside your plan for a completely full and independent review. It must also send it to the outside organization if it does not decide your appeal in the required time frames.

You must ask for your reconsideration within 60 days of the date of your "Notice of Denial of Medical Coverage." You should always file your request in writing.

Your appeal request should include your name, address, phone number, and your member identification number. Most importantly, state the reason for your appeal and attach any supporting information; it will be especially helpful to have a statement from your doctor or other medical documentation (e.g., progress notes, treatment orders). Clearly indicate why you do not agree with the plan's rationale in its "Notice of Denial of Medical Coverage" or its determination letter not to give you the care you want.

If there is no special urgency, you should ask for a standard or normal time reconsideration appeal. Your treating physician — that is, the one you have selected to give you the service — also has the right to request this standard time preservice reconsideration. Your plan must respond to the standard time first level appeals within 30 calendar days of its receipt of your appeal (with some exceptions).

Your standard time reconsideration request may have three possible results. The first is that your plan now decides that your reconsideration be granted in full, that is, completely in your favor. If so, it must authorize or provide the service you requested within 30 days of the date it first received the reconsideration (plus any time extension, if one was invoked). The second is that your plan decides not to grant your request in full; and the third is that it is unable to make a decision in the required time frame. In these cases, it must transfer your reconsideration to the outside Part C Qualified Independent Contractor (see section **3.1c**).

If by waiting up to 30 or possibly more days, you or your physician believes that your failure to get the service or services in a timely fashion will result in harm to your health or medical condition, then you should ask for a fast track, expedited, 72-hour appeal. In fact, if a physician says that your health would deteriorate if you don't get the service, your plan must fast-track the appeal. Note that any physician, not just your treating physician, may request this expedited time preservice reconsideration.

If only you (and not your physician) indicate this need for a fast track, your plan may or may not grant the need to expedite it, but it has only 72 hours to come to a conclusion on this issue. If, within that time frame, it says it will not expedite the decision but will stick to the standard 30-day track to make its reconsideration, you can grieve this decision, and your grievance has to be expedited.

To recap, your plan must give you its response as to whether your appeal will be expedited within 72 hours of its receipt of your request. Remember, the plan must actually notify you within these time frames, typically by calling you.

Your expedited reconsideration request will have the same three possible results as the standard reconsideration request, as discussed earlier. The only difference is that if your plan decides in your favor, you must get the service or treatment within 72 hours (rather than 30 days).

3.1c Transfer of cases to the Part C Qualified Independent Contractor

No matter which track you asked for, your plan has to either agree to provide the service which you requested, in which case your appeal was completely successful, or transfer your reconsideration to the outside Part C Qualified Independent Contractor. This is an outfit that is under contract with the Centers for Medicaid & Medicaid Services to resolve these types of cases. Your plan must also make this transfer if it does not make its decision in the time frames discussed in the previous sections.

When your plan deems that it cannot fully go along with your reconsideration request or cannot meet the deadlines, it must send your case file to this organization. It will notify you of this in writing, and its letter will tell you that the Part C Qualified Independent Contractor will be contacting you to see if you want to submit additional information. For example, additional information may be that you had more test results come in from a lab and you want to have these considered at this time.

The Part C Qualified Independent Contractor will also solicit any new information from you, and then proceed to complete the reconsideration. If it finds wholly or partly in your favor, that is, it decides that the service you wanted should completely or at least to some extent be given to you, your plan has set time frames to do so. If your request was decided on the standard time track, your plan has 14 days to provide the service to you. If it was decided on the fast track or expedited basis, your plan must authorize or provide the service within 72 hours of receiving the decision.

However, if the Part C Qualified Independent Contractor does not fully concur with your reconsideration request, it will inform you of this and indicate what your appeal rights are. From this point on your appeal process is the same as for all Medicare matters; see section 2.

3.2 Your basic right to a decision on a claim and how to appeal it

The previous sections explained the determination and appeal process for services and items that you have not actually received. This section discusses how to get your plan to cover a service that you have already received and that you believe it should pay for, or pay more than it says it should or has. This section will be particularly important to those of you in a plan such as a Private Fee-for-Service plan, in which you are basically responsible for arranging and getting your care, or possibly in a more structured plan in which you decide to use the point-of-service option.

These services will generally fall into several specific areas. One is when you may be traveling away from your plan's service area and you obtain medical treatment. Sometimes these treatments are fully anticipated, such as renal dialysis; at other times they are completely unexpected ones, such as a quick visit to a doctor because of the onset of some alarming symptoms.

Another is when you are in your plan's service area but get services in an out-of-network setting. For example, suppose you get transported to a hospital in the middle of the night by your local fire department following your 911 call reporting chest pains. They take you to a hospital whose emergency room physicians are not part of your plan's network. You can get covered in this situation.

A third situation emerges when you received services thinking everything was set with your plan but for some reason your plan doesn't want to pay now. For example, suppose a specialist's receptionist told you that your plan approved your visit, but now your plan says it did no such thing.

The fourth situation includes those times when you deliberately obtain a service when your plan refused to authorize it, but you believed it was important for your health. In effect, you bypassed the formal procedures outlined earlier, and took matters into your own hands. Or you didn't think the plan's doctor was the best one for you, and you went to one of your own choosing. This approach is a risky one, and generally not advised, but some beneficiaries have been known to do this when they believe their health is in real jeopardy, unless they get the care they choose, even when they know it is unauthorized.

3.2a Your right to a decision on a claim

The process you use to try and get your plan to pay a claim for an already delivered service follows much the same pattern as described in section 3.1 for getting a service, except there are no provisions for expedited decisions because it's a claim for a service that has already been done, not your health, which is now the issue.

The first thing you do is to get your plan to make a determination on your medical bill. You may already have this in the form of a letter or claim notice from your plan denying payment (if you do, skip to section 3.2b). If you don't, you need to submit a copy of the bill along with your request in writing for the plan to pay it or to reimburse you if you already paid it yourself. With this, you should give a detailed statement as to why you believe your plan should pay it.

Obviously, for more complex medical reasons, it would also be helpful for your claim to have a physician or health care provider support you with a statement or other medical documentation, and the more complex the issue, the more vital this would be.

You should mail this "request for a determination" to your plan, keeping a copy of everything. You can also present it in person. The plan has 60 calendar days from the day it receives your request to make a decision. If this decision is completely in your favor, and the plan pays, great! However, if the plan does not accept the claim in full, it must send you a "Notice of Denial of Payment," which explains why it will not pay, and which also tells you about appeal rights and how to exercise your rights.

3.2b Your appeal rights to reconsideration of a claim

The first-step appeal rights are your rights to a "reconsideration," although your notice may not specifically call it this. To exercise this appeal step, you must file within 60 calendar days of the date of the "Notice of Denial of Payment" you receive. You must do this in writing and tell your plan why you do not agree with its decision. Again, attach any documentation and keep copies of everything. You should send this return receipt requested, or in some way that you can ensure delivery is made and when.

Your plan will have 60 calendar days to make a decision on your appeal request. The plan can either find fully in your favor in this time frame, or it must forward your request to the Part C Qualified Independent Contractor.

The Qualified Independent Contractor will then make a decision on the appeal and send you and your plan a letter telling you what it is. If it is not fully in your favor, it will tell you in detail how you can appeal it. From this point on these appeals follow the steps for all Medicare appeals.

3.3 Right to file a grievance

Every Medicare managed care plan has to have a process to receive, examine, act on, and record any complaint or dispute you have with them. When you complain or initiate a dispute, you are technically making a grievance, which you have the right to file under Medicare law.

Just about anything can be a grievance. Typical examples are that you experience inappropriate demeanor or behavior by a plan employee, you can't get through on the phone, or you are unable to get an appointment at a reasonably convenient time.

You can file a grievance in person, over the phone, or in writing. Your plan's literature has the specific phone number and mailing address for these. Grievances have to be filed in 60 days of whatever action precipitate them. Plans have, under normal circumstances, 30 days to resolve the grievances. One important rule is that if the issue involves quality of care, the plan must respond to you in writing. The plan's response must also let you know of your right to file a formal complaint on quality of care with a Quality Improvement Organization.

3.4 Right to express dissatisfaction about quality of care

Quality Improvement Organizations are the bodies that the Medicare program uses to review formal complaints about quality of care. Note that the time frames and procedures that these organizations follow to review complaints coming from a Medicare Advantage enrollee are the same as those from a beneficiary in Original Medicare. However, the substance of the review differs.

Specifically, a Medicare Advantage enrollee's complaint is examined not only in terms of whether or not the quality of services "meet professionally recognized standards of health care," as all such complaints are. But because of the possibility of underutilization of services in the managed care setting, the Quality Improvement Organization also has to examine the complaint from three other points of view:

- Was the enrollee given appropriate services?

- Were these services given in an appropriate setting?

- Did the enrollee have access to adequate care?

This means that your managed care quality complaint will get looked at from several different angles.

4. Part D: Rights, Determinations, and Appeals

There is no separate section for Part D determinations and appeals for those of you in Original Medicare as opposed to those of you who have joined a Medicare Advantage Plan. This is

because the instructions are virtually the same for all beneficiaries. This section will use the term "drug plan" when referring to either your stand-alone drug plan or to your Medicare Advantage Plan, if you get your Part D prescription drug coverage from it.

In Part D when you get a prescription filled, the transaction is done electronically, up front, which is similar to using a credit card in which the merchant knows if the charge will be accepted before you get the merchandise. The pharmacy will know, before it actually dispenses your prescription, what the situation is, for example, that the medicine your doctor prescribed is not on your drug plan's formulary. Or it may even be that before you go to the pharmacy you know or your doctor knows that your drug plan won't pay for a particular drug.

Because of this, the Medicare law gives you and your physician the right to ask for an up-front exception to what your drug plan does not cover. It's almost like getting an "appeal" with the first decision. This exception process has three unique aspects of special benefit to you:

- It encompasses much more than just what is or is not on the formulary.

- Your drug plan must meet very strict time frames in which it must give you a decision about your request for an exception.

- If you don't get your decision in a timely fashion, your request automatically becomes an appeal, which partly explains why it's hard to separate the initial decision from the appeal.

For all the steps detailed in the following sections, either you, a representative you have appointed to act on your behalf, or those who have authority to act for you under law, typically state law, may take action. In addition, your prescribing physician may also take action, which is unusual in Medicare.

4.1 Your special rights under Part D

Beneficiaries and their doctors should clearly understand that they have powerful rights under the Part D law. While you have these special rights only with regard to what are called "coverage" decisions and appeals, these are fairly broad and are so very specifically defined and enumerated as to reinforce your rights. Moreover, one of these special rights is that you or your prescribing physician may request that your determination and appeal be "expedited," which requires your drug plan to respond swiftly to your request. This is in the law because decisions on what drugs your drug plan pays for can have immediate consequences to your health.

To exercise your special rights, you need to understand what Part D calls a "coverage determination" or coverage decision. In general, a coverage determination or decision is made when your drug plan will not furnish or pay for the specific prescription drug you or your doctor thinks you need, or it won't supply you with the dosage or quantities prescribed, or it wants to charge you too much to fill your prescription. More explicitly, the decision by the drug plan must be based on the following ten issues:

1. The drug is not legally covered under Part D of Medicare (i.e., the law excludes the drug from being paid for by this part of the program).

2. The prescription was furnished by an out-of-network pharmacy.

3. The amount of cost sharing you have to pay (i.e., the deductible, the coinsurance, or the co-payment you are responsible for) is incorrect or too high.

4. Medical necessity (i.e., your drug plan doesn't believe the drug is necessary for your medical condition).

The major coverage determinations may be problems with formulary issues, which include:

5. The drug you need is not on your drug plan's formulary (i.e., the plan's list of drugs it will pay for). Note that you can appeal a drug-not-on-formulary decision if your drug plan has been paying for the drug and then removes it from its formulary; or because it is not on the formulary, but your doctor now prescribes it; or when you join a plan and find out that your drug is not on its formulary.

6. Your drug is in a high-cost tier. That is, your drug plan will furnish the drug, but it will make you pay a higher-than-normal coinsurance or co-payment amount for it because you need that specific drug and no other drugs on a lower-cost tier are right for you. This is the same as saying your drug is not on the drug plan's preferred list for that class of medicine. Note that you can appeal a drug-in-a-high-cost-tier issue if your drug plan switches your drug from a regular- to a high-cost tier and you now have to pay more; or because it is in the high-cost tier when your doctor begins to prescribe it; or when you join a plan and find out that your drug is in a high-cost tier.

7. Your drug plan requires you to take step therapy (i.e., you have to first try a different medication other than that which was prescribed to see if that improves your medical condition).

8. Your drug plan requires you to undergo therapeutic substitution (i.e., the substitution of a prescribed drug by one that is not its generic equivalent).

9. Your drug plan restricts the number of pills or quantities you can have (i.e, it has dosage limitations).

When speed is important, number 10 applies:

10. A coverage determination includes the failure of the drug plan to notify you of a coverage decision within 72 hours of your request for a drug if your health would be adversely affected. You can appeal the lack of a timely determination in and of itself when that delay is harmful to your health or medical well-being.

You can see that you have some broad grounds to try to get your drug plan to fill your particular prescription and even to price it more favorably for you. Remember that you are generally not allowed to switch your drug plan except when the calendar year changes, so these procedures may come in very handy for you. Your attitude should be that in a case in which your condition, your health status, or your medical improvement genuinely need something other than what your drug plan offers, you ought to get it.

4.2 How to make a standard or normal time determination

You should use the standard or normal time procedures when a very quick decision is not needed. For example, you believe your drug plan overcharged you on a three-month mail-order prescription. You have the pills, so your health is good, but your pocketbook isn't.

If you want your drug plan to decide on any of the ten items mentioned in section **4.1**, you, your representative, or your prescribing physician, may make the request. The request may be made either by phone or in writing. The materials your drug plan sent you will give you the specific phone number and address for the request.

Your request should clearly state what you want that is different than what the drug plan would ordinarily provide, and the reasons. If any medical issue is involved, and it likely will be, it will be vital to have your physician to either make the request or to provide a statement supporting your request (this can be done by phone or in writing). In fact, if you want a decision on medical necessity or for one of the formulary issues (see section **4.1** numbers 5 through 9), you have to have such a statement, and in it your doctor must say why the prescription you need would either be more effective than the drug the drug plan wants to give you, or the plan's drug would have adverse effects on you, or both.

When your drug plan receives your request, it has 72 hours to respond, which it will usually do by phone. If its response is negative, it must also supply you with a written denial notice indicating its reasons and describing your appeal rights. At this point you can ask for a first step appeal — a redetermination. You can ask for the redetermination to be made on either a normal or an expedited basis.

If your drug plan does not give you a decision in 72 hours (remember this is not an expedited appeal), it must transfer your request to the Part D Qualified Independent Contractor, where your request automatically becomes a second-level appeal (i.e, a reconsideration, which means the decision is no longer in the hands of your drug plan).

4.2a How to make a standard or normal time redetermination appeal

If your drug plan's initial determination or decision is not completely in your favor, you have the right to appeal it. This first level of appeal is called a "redetermination," and it's done by your drug plan.

It should be clearly understood, if you originally asked for a standard or normal time determination, you don't have to stay on that track. Therefore, if your condition has worsened, or if other circumstances require the prompt start of a particular medication, you may now file for an expedited redetermination (see section **4.3b**).

The drug plan's written determination denial notice must explain to you in detail how to make this standard time redetermination appeal. Your drug plan may, at its option, take oral requests. The best advice is to always file your requests in writing and keep copies of everything you submit. (Of course, you can consider faxing or emailing to ensure the drug plan gets your request promptly.) You must file for your request within 60 calendar days of the date on the notice of decision you received.

Follow the advice in section **4.2** on "standard determinations" on what to include in your appeal and include any information on how your condition may have changed. As always, your prescribing physician's statement will be key, so be certain to submit it with your appeal. However, your prescribing physician cannot make this appeal on his or her own.

Once filed, your drug plan has only seven calendar days from when it received your appeal request to respond to you, and it must always respond to you in writing. As with your initial determination request, its response must also indicate, if its redetermination is not wholly favorable to you, what its reasons are, what your next appeal step is, and how to take it.

If your drug plan does not send you a decision in seven calendar days, it must transfer your request to the Part D Qualified Independent Contractor, at which time your redetermination request automatically becomes a second-level appeal (i.e., a reconsideration).

4.3 Expedited procedures

You should use the expedited time process whenever your current medical condition, or the possibility that it might deteriorate, requires you to have a drug, or a dosage level, or any exception, to what your drug plan wants to give you. As can be seen in the following sections, decision times for these requests are considerably faster than those required of drug plans for the standard time procedures described in the previous two sections.

4.3a How to make an expedited determination request

The same requirements and procedures outlined in section **4.2** for a standard time determination request also apply here with one additional item: You must tell your drug plan why an immediate, expedited determination is appropriate. If your prescribing physician submits a statement that an expedited request is necessary to prevent serious jeopardy to your life, your health, or your ability to recover maximum function, your drug plan must expedite your determination.

Keep in mind that there are two decision points on your expedited request. First, whether your request will be expedited and, second, what the plan's determination is on whether you should get the drug or dosage or whatever you believe you should have. There are three possible outcomes for an expedited determination request (unless otherwise indicated, the following time frames are counted from when your drug plan receives your request):

1. Within 24 hours, the drug plan both grants that a quick decision is appropriate, and it makes that decision or determination, and notifies you by phone. The determination may be in your favor, or not. If it is not, you may appeal it.

2. Within 24 hours the drug plan first concludes that a quick decision is not needed; and then, within a total of 72 hours, it makes its actual decision or determination, and notifies you by phone. The determination may be in your favor, or not. You may grieve the first conclusion. If the determination is not in your favor, you may appeal it.

- If the first part of scenario number 2 happens (i.e., the drug plan decides within 24 hours that it should not expedite your request), it must notify you by phone and you may file a grievance about this issue. You may do this immediately, by phone. This may prod the drug plan into a quick decision; in any case, it must respond to your grievance within 24 hours of its receipt. In effect, you get two chances to get your request expedited. If your grievance is approved, that is, the drug plan now decides that you should get an expedited decision, it has to make that decision within 24 hours of this approval.

3. Neither 1 nor 2 occurs. In this case, your drug plan has decided within 24 hours to give or not give an expedited decision, but has not made the actual determination in the time frames shown in numbers 1 and 2 (i.e., within those 24 hours when it agrees that an expedited determination is appropriate, or within 72 hours when it does not agree). In these cases, your drug plan has a total of 48 hours, or 96 hours respectively, to transfer your determination request to the Qualified Independent Contractor, at which time it automatically becomes a second-level appeal or reconsideration.

Note that if either scenario 1 or 2 occurs, and the drug plan's actual determination is not wholly favorable to you, then it has three calendar days after it tells you of its determination to send you a written notice of it.

4.3b How to make an expedited redetermination appeal

If your drug plan's actual determination or decision is not wholly in your favor, which can happen in either the standard or the expedited determination process, you have the right to appeal that determination. You can ask that this first-level appeal or redetermination be expedited, whether or not you asked for an expedited determination. This first-level appeal is called a "redetermination," and it's done by your drug plan. You must file for this within 60 calendar days of the date on the written notice of the decision you received.

Use the information presented in section **4.3a** in asking for an initial determination and indicate why it should be expedited. If your prescribing physician submits the statement described there, your drug plan must expedite your redetermination request. This process works much like the initial expedited determination process, but the time frames are slightly longer.

You, or your prescribing physician, may file your expedited redetermination request. It can be made either orally or in writing, and your written determination letter from your drug plan will give details on how to do this. Again, the best advice is that since you are clearly in disagreement with your drug plan, you should file your request in writing; your drug plan will give you a number where you can fax it. Your appeal should clearly state why you believe the drug plan's determination is not correct; include any information that was not considered by the plan (e.g., specifics about your condition or how it has changed). Include your prescribing physician's statement; again, your doctor can give this over the phone or in writing. Also, tell your drug plan why an immediate, expedited redetermination is appropriate.

Importantly, just as with an initial determination, if your prescribing physician submits a statement that an expedited redetermination is necessary to prevent serious jeopardy to your life, your health, or your ability to recover maximum function, your drug plan must expedite it.

There are three possible outcomes for an expedited redetermination request, and they follow the same three outcomes outlined in section 4.3a for an expedited determination request except some of the time frames are slightly different:

1. Within 72 hours, your drug plan grants that a quick appeal decision is appropriate, and it makes that redetermination. If not wholly favorable to you, you can appeal.

2. The drug plan does two things: First, it decides that a quick appeals decision is not needed and notifies you of this, all within 24 hours. (You may grieve this, and do so immediately by phone.) Second, it then makes its redetermination, and orally notifies you of it, both within seven days. Again, if not wholly favorable, you can appeal.

3. Neither of the two options above occurs. The drug plan has a total of 24 additional hours to transfer your request to the Part D Qualified Independent Contractor. (These 24 hours are added either to the 72 hours in scenario 1 or the seven days in scenario 2.)

4.4 Second level appeals: Reconsiderations

If the actual redetermination is not wholly in your favor, you have the right to appeal further.

This second-level appeal is called a "reconsideration," and you always have the right to request this on an expedited basis. Your notice from your drug plan will tell you how to file this appeal to the Part D Qualified Independent Contractor.

4.4a How to make a standard or normal time reconsideration appeal

You or your representative must file your reconsideration appeal request in writing, and you must do so within 60 days of the notice of redetermination. Your physician cannot file for you. There is no special form or format to use. Your written redetermination letter from your drug plan will also give details on how to do this. Your appeal should clearly state why you believe the drug plan's redetermination is not correct, and should include any new information, such as additional specifics about why your condition has changed.

Be sure to keep copies of everything you file. Once the Qualified Independent Contractor receives your standard reconsideration appeal, it has seven days to make its decision, which it must do in writing.

4.4b How to make an expedited reconsideration appeal

If you want your reconsideration expedited, be sure to specify this, and include your reasons. Also, if there is even more urgency for speed because of deterioration in your condition, emphasize that. Once the Qualified Independent Contractor receives your expedited reconsideration appeal, it has 72 hours to make its decision, which it must do in writing. No matter which time track you filed your appeal on, the Qualified Independent Contractor, if it finds wholly or partly in your favor, it will inform you and your drug plan of its reconsideration appeal decision. This decision is completely binding on your plan.

If the Qualified Independent Contractor does not find wholly in your favor, it will tell you in writing, and it will also tell you your appeal rights.

4.5 Subsequent appeals

From this point on, your appeal rights are the same as with all other Parts of Medicare, which begins in section **2.4**. The only special item concerns how the amount in controversy is calculated in Part D. Because you enroll in a drug plan on a year-to-year basis, it is calculated the same way. For example, if your dispute with your drug plan began in July, and it's now December, and you think you should have a maintenance drug with a co-payment of $20 per month and your drug plan says it should be a co-payment of $50, the amount in controversy is $180 (six months times the $30 monthly difference).

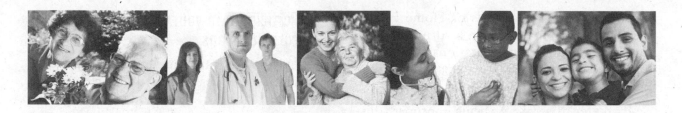

15
Your Rights as a Medicare Beneficiary: Know Them and Use Them!

As a beneficiary of the Medicare program, you are surrounded with powerful and extensive protections and rights under federal law. This chapter will discuss the more general rights that all beneficiaries have under the program as well as specific rights that you have if you are in Original Medicare.

This chapter will also discuss your privacy rights. While these are the same for both Original Medicare and Medicare Advantage beneficiaries, they are distinct rights, and are a little different because the Medicare program itself is subject to them, as well as to the health care delivery system in which you actually get your care.

Along with rights come responsibilities, and you do have responsibilities to the Medicare program. Medicare is your program, and you need to support and sustain it as appropriate.

1. Entitlement and Enrollment Rights for Medicare Applicants and Beneficiaries

You have extensive appeal rights regarding your entitlement to Part A and Part B of Medicare,

and to the amounts of your premiums, which were discussed in previous chapters.

Note, however, that you do not have any appeal rights to your enrollment to Part C or to Part D (other than Part D's extra help). If you request to join a Part C Medicare Advantage or managed care plan or a Part D drug plan is denied, you are told to contact the customer service department of the plan you tried to join to solve the problem. The same is true if you think you should have an earlier or different effective date of enrollment, or what the penalty amount of your Part D premium should be. If you cannot resolve it with your plan, you should immediately contact the Centers for Medicare & Medicaid in lieu of any formal appeals rights.

1.1 Be protected against discrimination

You are protected against discrimination based on your race, color, national origin, ethnicity, religion, creed, disability, sex, handicap, sexual orientation, or age.

All participants in the Medicare program, whether they are individual practitioners such as physicians; or groups such as clinics; or institutions such as hospitals or Home Health Agencies; or companies such as drug plans or Medicare Advantage organizations, are simply prohibited under federal law to discriminate for the above listed reasons.

If you feel that you are being improperly discriminated against, you can either discuss it with the party involved, or you can bring a complaint to the Office of Civil Rights of the US Department of Health and Human Services. These are the people who are specifically designated to handle these types of complaints by Medicare beneficiaries. This office also has the responsibility for enforcing those rights. Contacts for this office's central and regional offices are included in the Resources section on the CD.

1.2 Receive services in a culturally competent way

You have the right to receive services in a culturally competent way. As part of, or an extension of this, you have the right to get health-care services in a language you can understand and in a culturally sensitive way. Talk to your provider if you think this is an issue. You can always discuss it with the Office of Civil Rights.

This right may be more important to those beneficiaries in a Medicare Advantage or managed care plan that have a restricted network, as their choice of providers may not be as varied as they might wish.

1.3 Get information from Medicare

You have the legal right to receive the *Medicare & You* handbook when you first join Medicare and each year thereafter as well as the right to access the Medicare toll-free phone number. These are your statutory rights, not just things the program does to help communicate with you.

1.4 Participate in your health care decisions

Not only do you have the right to participate in making all your health-care decisions, but you also have the right of having others such as family members help you make decisions about your health care.

1.5 Advance notice for proposed medical care or treatment that is part of a research experiment

Not only must you be told about any research being conducted with your care or treatment, but you must be given the choice of refusing experimental treatments.

1.6 Use advance directives

Advance directives are written documents that say ahead of time how you want medical decisions about end-of-life care to be made in case you are unable to do so by yourself. They include living wills, durable powers of attorney, health care proxies, and do-not-resuscitate orders. Too few beneficiaries have these. You should be aware that although there are federal statutes concerning these, state laws determine their content and validity, and it's absolutely essential to deal with an attorney in your state. Thus you may also wish to contact your State Health Insurance Assistance Program (SHIP) for additional information or referral to an eldercare legal contact, or call your state or local bar association for further direction.

1.7 File a complaint about the quality of your care

You have the right to file a complaint about the quality of care you are receiving or have received.

You may file a formal quality of care complaint with the Medicare Quality Improvement Organization (QIO) that serves your area. These are the bodies that the Medicare program has given the responsibility to review formal complaints about quality of care, particularly when the issue surrounds the care given or directed by a health care practitioner, and especially by a physician. They review quality of care complaints fairly rapidly (i.e., within three days) if the Medicare beneficiary is still in a facility or actually receiving services, but quite slowly when this is not the case.

All these complaints must be filed in writing, but you can call the Quality Improvement Organization and get them put your complaint in writing for your signature. You will be asked whether or not you consent to their revealing your identity in the course of their review. If you refuse to allow this, in many cases the review will not proceed. The information these outfits gather is privileged, and is generally not releasable under law. The thinking is that unless the information is kept strictly confidential, no one will cooperate with the Quality Improvement Organization's fact finding and review process. Their basic aim is not to punish or discipline, but to improve quality of care through an educational and instructional process.

Not all quality of care issues are reviewed by the Quality Improvement Organizations. Where a health care facility is involved, and that facility is certified as provider in the Medicare program, your complaint may be reviewed by a State Survey Agency. These certified facilities include:

- Hospitals
- Skilled Nursing Facilities
- Home Health Agencies
- End-Stage Renal Disease Dialysis Centers
- Comprehensive Outpatient Rehab Facilities
- Community Mental Health Centers
- Religious Non-Medical Health Care Institutions
- Rural health clinics
- Federally Qualified Health Centers
- Ambulatory Surgical Centers
- Clinical laboratories
- Portable X-ray suppliers
- Hospices
- Nursing homes

State Survey Agencies are entities within your state government, often part of a larger department of health or some such cabinet-level outfit, which has an agreement with the federal government to make sure that these facilities meet Medicare standards (i.e., they may be certified as participating in Medicare). While the majority of the inspections these agencies perform involve nursing homes, they will get involved with your complaint particularly if it involves an institutional issue regarding care, and not just a practitioner one. For example, if you were being treated and a medical machine malfunctioned; or you were exposed to an unsafe condition in an operating room; or your requests for help given on your call button were not answered; or you developed a nosocomial infection while an inpatient; or a lab mixed up test results: These are the kinds of quality of care issues these agencies investigate.

Unlike complaints made to Quality Improvement Organizations, these do not have to be in writing, but you will get a response in writing. This response will include information about what method the agency used to conduct its investigation, when it was conducted, its overall conclusion about your complaint, a summary of its findings, and an indication of what action it has taken or will take.

Note that Medicare does not pay for routine nursing home stays, as discussed in Chapter 2, and the vast majority of complaints these agencies get concern nursing homes, so if you are or a loved one is in a nursing home, and there is a problem, these agencies will investigate it no matter who is paying for or covering the person's care.

It may take some time for you to get a response, as these agencies' staffs are limited, and they have a fairly rigid prioritization system to insure that the most vital complaints are handled first. If the agency thinks a patient is in danger, it will react very quickly.

Finally, know that the agencies will not investigate all of your complaints. Some complaints are of such a serious nature that the agency will refer them directly to the Centers for Medicare & Medicaid Services for a federal investigation. If a hospital or other provider is accredited by a federally recognized accrediting organization, such as the Joint Commission, and the substance of the complaint is not highly serious, it may refer the complaint to that organization for its review.

2. Your Beneficiary Rights in Original Medicare

2.1 Free choice by patient and provider

Unless you are in a Part D drug plan, all of which have designated pharmacies, you, as an Original Medicare beneficiary, can go to any provider that is qualified under Medicare and is willing to take you as a patient. You should understand that a provider does *not* have to treat you because it can choose whom it serves, subject to the previously mentioned rights and protections

you have under the antidiscrimination portions of the law.

2.2 Obtain an itemized statement

Obtaining an itemized statement is sort of an odd right, but the law is very clear about it. It was originally enacted as a protection against incorrect, improper, or fraudulent billing, so that you, as a health care consumer, could get detailed information about a medical bill if you wanted it. For example, you thought you were overcharged. More recently this right has been emphasized as part of the attempt to get beneficiaries involved in antifraud activities to help safeguard the program.

You have the right to request an itemized statement from any entity that provided you with a service or item that the Medicare program paid for. Your request must be in writing and the entity must respond in 30 days. If it does not respond in 30 days, you have the right to request, in writing, that the Centers for Medicare & Medicaid Services obtain it from the provider.

When you get the statement, you also have the right, within 90 calendar days, to have Centers for Medicare & Medicaid Services review it, if you believe you were overcharged, or not given a service as claimed, or were billed twice (duplicate billing). If Medicare confirms any irregularity, it can recover any improper payments it made to the provider.

You could use this right if you need an itemized statement to file a third-party claim and your provider is unwilling to give you this information.

3. Your Rights to Privacy Protections

In the Medicare system, information about you is passed back and forth between many entities for a whole variety of purposes. A few reasons for the transfer of your information would include entitling and enrolling you in the various parts of Medicare; establishing your eligibility for special programs such as extra help; billing you for premiums you may owe, which may include checking your income tax returns; reviewing information about your health status when you join a managed care organization; collecting information on what other insurance you may have; reviewing the quality of care given by institutions and individual practitioners; and responding to your inquiries.

A number of federal entities are included, such as the Centers for Medicare & Medicaid Services and the Social Security Administration, but there are others, including the US Department of Health and Human Services' Inspector General and the US Department of Justice. Also some state agencies use your personal Medicare information including your State Survey Agency, which inspects a variety of health care institutions. Also, the Medicare program contracts out almost all of its day-to-day work of claims processing, computer operations, systems programming, quality review, fraud analysis, and inquiry response to dozens of private companies, all of which use or handle data about you.

The following list will help you understand what your rights are to privacy protections:

- You have the right to require the government to keep your Medicare information private and safeguarded so it isn't illegally released or revealed.

- You have the right to view and get a copy of any personal medical information that Medicare has in its possession about you.

- If you believe that the personal health information Medicare possesses about you is incorrect, or that it is missing something, you have the right to ask that your information be corrected or amended. If Medicare does not agree, you have the right

to have your statement of disagreement appended to your record.

- You have the right to get a list of people or institutions who were given your health care information, if it was not a routine operational disclosure. (These routine disclosures include passing information about you to a Medicare Administrative Contractor to process a claim, or if law enforcement is involved, giving them claims information about you as maybe a health care provider you used is being investigated by the Inspector General or the Federal Bureau of Investigation.)

- You have a right to ask Medicare to communicate to you in a different manner or at a different place. For example, to change your address to a different one if you don't want people at your current delivery place to know that you are getting material from Medicare.

- You can restrict your information in some cases. If Medicare wants to give out information about you that is not in its Privacy Notice, Medicare must ask your written permission to do so. You have the right to give this permission or not and, if you give it, to revoke it at will.

- You always have the right to ask Medicare not to give out information about you. It may or may not accede to your request.

4. Your Responsibilities

Beneficiaries have two serious responsibilities when it comes to using the benefits provided by Medicare. One is to guard against overutilization; the other is to help safeguard the program against fraud and abuse.

With regard to overutilization, beneficiaries need to realize that to a degree they control how many services Medicare pays for. No doubt there is tremendous overutilization of Medicare services. As a patient and as a beneficiary you need to be willing to question the need for the frequency of visits to your doctor, or to repeat tests, or even get a test that won't change how you are being treated.

It is also your responsibility to safeguard against fraud and abuse. The worst frauds are when Medicare beneficiaries are given treatments that harm their health, or even lulled into thinking they are being properly treated for a disease when they are not. It's not just money, it's your health, and your life, too. Read over the following list to help protect yourself from fraud and abuse:

- Protect your Medicare number as much as you do your Social Security number and treat both of them like a checking account or credit card number. Don't give these numbers to anyone over the phone or in person, unless you initiated the contact and you know to whom you are talking. Don't leave your Medicare number on a phone message. Don't accept any gift or offer of free services or supplies in return for your Medicare number. In fact, don't carry your Medicare number with you unless you are going to get a medical service and will need it.

- Don't allow anyone else to use your Medicare number or card, Medicare Advantage member card, or Part D drug plan card.

- Don't ask your doctor to order a service, test, supply, or prescription on your behalf unless you really need it. Certainly don't ask him or her to falsify entries such as diagnoses on bills or certificates of need, or on your records, in order to get Medicare to pay or approve anything.

- Don't allow anyone, except your physician or a medical professional known to you or involved in your care, to review your medical records, or to recommend medical services or supplies for you.

- Never deal with people who show up at your door and claim they represent the Medicare program, or the Medicare branch of the federal government, or are "sent by the government." If they are at your door, slam it and call the police; the police can verify their identity.

- Remember that Medicare does not sell anything. If anyone tells you that "Medicare wants you to have" a medical supply, exam, or service, they are ripping you off.

- If a provider routinely waives coinsurance or co-payments on any Medicare supply or service that should be charged, without genuinely checking on your ability to pay, it's a scam. Or if you challenge having to pay coinsurance, and they quickly say "don't worry about it, we'll take care of it," it's a scam.

- No reputable provider will ever use high pressure or scare tactics to sell you any medical supply or service or diagnostic test. Hang up on telemarketers. Slam the door on door-to-door salespeople and, again, call the police.